$5.99

MW01592151

# Table of Contents

# INTRODUCTION

Ketogenic Diet is a diet comprising of low-carbohydrate, sufficient-protein and high-fat. The type of diet enables the body to burn fat instead of carbohydrates and helps a lot in weight loss.

## Importance of Ketogenic Diet

Ketogenic diet has an important role in medical science as it is used as a cure for epilepsy in children. Glucose & insulin are produced by taking high amount of carbohydrates. These carbohydrates transform into glucose and are utilized in stimulating brain-functioning. High carbohydrates force the human body to utilize glucose as the main source of energy, leading into fat storage in the body. Conversion of fat into ketone bodies and fatty acids happens if the quantity of carbohydrates is lower in diet. Glucose is used as the prime energy source when these ketone bodies reach the brain.

In case of low food consumption, the body naturally initiates the process of ketosis. The aim of having a ketogenic diet is to enable your body into a metabolic state that it burns fat. Lowering the carbohydrates & excess of fats, ketones will act as the key source of energy for the body.

## Advantages of Ketogenic Diet

1. Contributions to Weight loss
2. Enhanced Mental Focus
3. For Treatment of Epilepsy
4. Acne Treatment

5. Optimization of Insulin

## Ketogenic Diet Tips

Ketogenic diet is beneficial in weight loss, enhancing energy levels and eliminates the threat of certain diseases.

1. Irregular Fasting
2. Regular Exercise
3. Low Protein Intake
4. Improve Sleep
5. Proper Water Intake
6. High Salt consumption
7. Opt Carbohydrates Wisely
8. Less Stress

## Food consumptions:

**Dos**: Foods like spinach (leafy greens), cheese, butter (High Fat Dairy), raspberries, eat nuts & broccoli, etc. should be consumed.

**Don'ts**: Foods like corn, rice (grains), fruits, honey (sugar) etc. should be avoided.

## Slow Cooker:

Conventional cooking has taken a new turn with the advent of the slow cooker. It can assist you in everyday cooking involving any ingredient from any food category. To explain how beneficial slow cooking is and what draw backs it has, following will help you on getting answers to these questions.

## Advantages:

**1. Energy Saver:**

In comparison to other coking appliances like ovens etc, the slow cooker utilizes lesser amount of power and doesn't waste any energy at all.

**2. User Friendly:**

It is very convenient in usage and proves to be extremely user friendly. Just gather the ingredients and have your lunch in a short time.

**3. Odorless:**

There is absolutely no smell coming out of the slow cooker unless someone manually opens the lid. This may not be appreciated as this may increase the time of cooking.

**4. No burning:**

Foods like meat can be cooked for a longer time in a slow cooker, the might get dry because of longer cooking time but there is no chance of burning at all.

## Disadvantages:

1. Incompatible with canned foods
2. Slow cooking time
3. Takes a lot in preparations and planning
4. Loss of Nutrients
5. Bean toxins

# Breakfast

## Mushroom Casserole

**Serves: 8**

**Prep Time: 30 mins**

The slow cooker mushroom casserole is a unique savoury blend of eggs with cheese, cauliflower, and juicy leeks. The protein-rich sausages are there to boost you up for a day full of energy. It can be best served with warm bread or crispy toasts along with a refreshing smoothie of your choice.

### Ingredients

- 6 eggs
- 10 oz. cauliflower florets, diced
- 1/2 tsp salt
- Black pepper to taste
- 5 oz. cremini mushrooms, finely diced
- 12 fully cooked sausage links, cut into quarter-inch rounds
- 1 leek, cleaned and cut into quarter-inch half-moon slices
- 1 (8 oz.) package of Sargento sharp cheddar fine cut cheese

### Directions

1. Grease the base of your slow cooker with cooking spray.
2. Place pieces of cauliflower in a microwave-safe bowl and season them with ¼ tsp. salt.
3. Fill this bowl with water and microwave it for about 8 minutes.
4. Strain the cooked cauliflower and add them to the slow cooker.
5. Top the cauliflower pieces with sausage and mushrooms.
6. Whisk eggs with ¼ tsp. of salt in a bowl and stir in leeks and half of the cheese.

7. Pour this eggs mixture over the mushrooms in the slow cooker and cook for 2 to 3 hours on High.
8. Once done, top the casserole with remaining cheese, salt and pepper. Let it rest for 5 minutes.
9. Slice and serve.

## Nutrition

Calories: 244

Fats: 17.9g

Sodium: 534mg

Carbs: 5.4g

Proteins: 16.3g

Sugar: 1.8g

# Slow Cooker Breakfast Frittata

**Serves: 1**

**Prep Time: 5mins**

Frittatas are a morning delight when served fresh with steaming toasts. With the freshness of spinach, bel and seasoned eggs, this breakfast frittata is one scrumptious and healthy meal for you and your family.

## Ingredients

- ¾ cups drain spinach, frozen
- 1 ½ cups diced bell pepper, red
- ¼ cups diced onion, red
- 8 individual beat egg
- ½ teaspoons black pepper
- 1 teaspoon sea salt
- 1 ⅓ cups cook sausage, breakfast

## Directions

1. Add all the ingredients to a bowl and mix well to combine.
2. Pour this mixture into a well-greased slow cooker.
3. Cook for about 2 to 3 hours on Low.
4. Once done, slice the frittata into small pieces.
5. Serve warm or preserve for later use.

## Nutrition

Calories: 238

Fats: 16g

Sodium: 844mg

Carbs: 3g

Proteins: 20g

Sugar: 2g

# Mexican Casserole

**Serves: 10**

**Prep Time: 15mins**

Add savoury twist to the traditional egg casserole with Mexican salsa, milk and cheese. Rich and delicious spices like cumin and coriander are incorporated into the recipe to give a nice aromatic flavour to the eggs and sausages.

## Ingredients

- 12 ounces Jones Dairy Farm Pork Sausage Roll
- 1/2 teaspoon garlic powder
- 1/2 teaspoon coriander
- 1 teaspoon cumin1 teaspoon chilli powder
- 1/4 teaspoon salt
- 1/4 teaspoon pepper
- 1 cup salsa
- 10 eggs
- 1 cup milk
- 1 cup Pepper Jack cheese or cheese of choice

## Directions

1. Sauté pork sausage in a skillet over medium heat until it is no longer pink.
2. Season the sausages with salsa and all the remaining spices. Set it aside.
3. Whisk eggs with milk in separate bowl and stir in pork mixture along with cheese.
4. Grease the base of your slow cooker with cooking spray.
5. Pour the eggs mixture into the slow cooker and cook for 2 ½ hours on High.

6. Once done, serve the casserole with desired toppings and enjoy.

**Nutrition**

Calories: 320

Carbs: 5.2g

Fats: 24.1g

Proteins: 17.9g

Sodium: 749mg

Sugar: 1.6g

# Morning Quiche

**Serves: 8**

**Prep Time:   10mins**

Here is one healthy, creamy and rich in protein morning quiche which is loaded with delicious cheddar cheese and crispy cooked bacon. Spinach is added to give a healthy twist to the recipe and boost up its iron contents and various other essential minerals.

## Ingredients

- 1 tablespoon butter
- 10 eggs, beaten
- 1 cup light cream or half & half
- 8 ounces shredded cheddar cheese
- 1/2 teaspoon black pepper
- 10 pieces cooked bacon, chopped
- 1/2 cup chopped spinach (optional)

## Directions

1. Grease the base of your slow cooker with butter. Keep it aside
2. Mix all the ingredients in a bowl except bacon and pour this mixture into the cooker.
3. Top the mixture with bacon pieces and cover the lid.
4. Cook for about 4 hours on Low.
5. Avoid overcooking and remove the quiche from the cooker once done.
6. Serve warm.

## Nutrition

Calories: 303          Fats: 24.7g          Sodium: 655mg

Carbs: 1.4g          Proteins: 18.6g          Sugar: 0.5g

# Sweet Pepper Hash

**Serves: 10**

**Prep Time: 20mins**

Sweet pepper is famous for its mild tangy taste but when it is mixed with juicy sautéed onions, crispy sausages, dried herbs and eggs, its taste becomes irresistible. The sweet pepper hash is not only rich in protein but the addition of cheese makes it even healthier and appealing.

## Ingredients

- 12-ounce package cooked smoked chicken sausage with apple, quartered lengthwise and cut into 1/2-inch pieces
- 1 teaspoon olive oil
- 1 ½ cups sliced sweet onion
- 2 teaspoons snipped fresh thyme or 1/2 teaspoon dried thyme, crushed
- ½ teaspoon ground black pepper
- 10 eggs, beaten
- ¼ cup reduced-sodium chicken broth
- 1 ½ cups chopped green, red, and/or yellow sweet peppers
- ½ cup shredded Swiss cheese (2 ounces) (optional)
- 2 teaspoons snipped fresh tarragon or parsley
- ¼ cup shredded cheddar cheese

## Directions

1. Sauté sausages in a large skillet over medium heat for about 5 minutes.
2. Transfer the sausage to a plate and add onions to the same skillet. Cook for about 5 minutes.
3. Grease the base of the slow cooker with cooking spray.

4. Add browned sausage, sautéed onions, thyme, sweet pepper and black pepper to the cooker.
5. Whisk eggs with broth and pour this mixture over the vegetables in the cooker.
6. Cover the lid and cook for about 2 to 3 hours on High heat.
7. Top it with cheeses and allow it to melt.
8. Drizzle some tarragon on top and serve.

## Nutrition

Calories: 179

Fats: 11.6g

Sodium: 249mg

Carbs: 5.4g

Proteins: 12.6g

Sugar: 1.4g

# Grain-Free Granola with Orange Zest

**Serves: 20**

**Prep Time: 5mins**

Have a crunchy, juicy and healthy morning breakfast with this gluten free granola recipe which is extremely easy and quick to prepare. Once you add all the ingredients to the slow cooker, set it on high and ready to enjoy the scrumptious mixture of coconut shreds and delicious seeds.

## Ingredients

- 2 cups desiccated/shredded coconut unsweetened
- 1/4 cup sunflower seeds
- 1/4 cup pumpkin seeds
- 2/3 cup almonds chopped
- 2 tablespoons cacao nibs
- 3 tablespoons coconut oil
- 2 tablespoons granulated sweetener of choice or more, to taste
- 4 tablespoons cocoa powder unsweetened
- 2 tablespoons orange zest

## Directions

1. Add all the ingredients to the slow cooker and mix them well.
2. Cook for 4 hours on High and stir the mixture after every 15 minutes.
3. Once done, stir well and transfer to a serving plate.
4. Serve and enjoy.

## Nutrition

Calories: 277

Carbs: 9g

Fats: 26g

Proteins: 4.8g

Sodium: 249mg

Sugar: 2.2g

# Thai Slow Cooker Zucchini Lasagna

**Serves: 8**

**Prep Time: 45mins**

A zucchini rich morning lasagna is all what you need to start your day. It has the blend of delicious turkey ground, baked zucchini, cabbage, cheese and mouthwatering spices. When slow cooked together, these ingredients give a filling flavor which extends through all its layers.

## Ingredients

For the zoodles:

- 4 Large Zucchinis
- 1 Tablespoon Salt

For the lasagna:

- 2 Tablespoon Coconut oil
- 1 Pound Extra-lean ground turkey
- 1 Cup Onion, diced
- 1 Tablespoon 2 tsp Fresh garlic, minced, divided
- 1/2 Tablespoon Fresh ginger, minced
- Pepper
- 1 Cup Light coconut milk
- 1/4 Cup Natural creamy peanut butter
- 1/4 Cup Reduced sodium soy sauce
- 2 Tablespoon Coconut sugar
- 1 Tablespoon Rice vinegar
- 1 Tablespoon Fresh lime juice
- 1 Tablespoon Fish sauce
- 1-2 Tablespoon Sriracha
- 15 Oz Light ricotta cheese
- 1 Large Egg

- 1/2 Cup Cilantro, roughly chopped
- 2 Cups Nappa cabbage, roughly chopped
- 1/2 Cup Water chestnuts, diced
- 8 Ounces Mozzarella cheese, grated (about 2 tightly packed cups)
- 1 Large Red pepper, diced

For garnish:
- Cilantro, diced
- Green onion, diced
- Roasted peanuts, diced
- Bean sprouts, roughly chopped

## Directions

1. Preheat your oven to 350 F.
2. Slice the zucchini into 1/8 inch thick slices and spread the slices over 2 cookie sheets. Sprinkle a tablespoon of salt on top.
3. Bake the zucchini slices for 15 to 20 minutes.
4. Meanwhile, heat oil in a large skillet over medium heat. Sauté turkey ground, ginger, garlic and onion in the oil for about 10 to 12 minutes.
5. Stir in peanut butter, coconut milk, coconut sugar, soy sauce, rice vinegar, lime juice, 1 tablespoon Sriracha and fish sauce.
6. Bring this mixture to a boil for 3 minutes with constant stirring. Reduce the heat and let the mixture simmer for 2 to 4 minutes until it is creamy and thick.
7. Adjust seasoning as per taste then keep the mixture aside.
8. Once the zucchini is baked, transfer them onto a paper towel to absorb the excess moisture. Keep it aside.

9. Beat ricotta cheese with egg and a pinch of pepper in a bowl. Keep the mixture aside.

10. Grease the base of a 7 quart slow cooker and spread half of the turkey mixture in the cooker.

11. Top this mixture with zucchini noodles then a layer of half of the ricotta mixture.

12. Drizzle half of the cilantro then add half of the cabbage, half of the water chestnuts and half of the mozzarella cheese.

13. Repeat the layers in the same order using the remaining ingredients and top it with red pepper.

14. Cover the cooker and cook for about 4 to 5 hours on Low.

15. Once done, slice and serve warm.

## Nutrition

Calories: 341

Fats: 17.1g

Sodium: 1634mg

Carbs: 15.5g

Proteins: 31.2g

Sugar: 7.6g

# Mediterranean Frittata

**Serves: 10**

**Prep Time: 20mins**

Unlike traditional frittata recipe, this Mediterranean cuisine has a twist of oregano, arugula, roasted red peppers and delicious goat cheese. Once cooked, the frittata can be preserved in the refrigerator for about 2 days and reheat at low temperature before serving. Serve with crispy toasts for best flavor.

## Ingredients

- 8 eggs
- ⅓ cup milk
- 1 teaspoon dried oregano
- Salt and freshly ground black pepper, to taste
- 4 cups baby arugula
- 1¼ cups chopped roasted red peppers
- ½ cup thinly sliced red onion
- ¾ cup crumbled goat cheese

## Directions

1. Grease your slow cooker with nonstick spray.
2. Whisk eggs in a large bowl along with milk and oregano. Season the mixture with salt and pepper.
3. Spread baby arugula in the cooker and top it with roasted red peppers, red onion and goat cheese.
4. Top these layers with eggs mixture.
5. Cover and cook on low for about 2½ to 3 hours.
6. Serve and enjoy.

## Nutrition

Calories: 164

Carbs: 4g

Fats: 11g

Proteins: 12g

Sodium: 249mg

Sugar: 3g

# Zucchini Bread

**Serves: 12**

**Prep Time: 10mins**

This bread is a good low carb alternative which is filled with savory zucchini shreds and vanilla. The simple blend of basic bread ingredients with a crunchy twist of walnuts gives this bread a refreshing flavor for a morning meal.

## Ingredients

- 1 cup almond flour
- 1/3 cup coconut flour
- 2 teaspoons cinnamon
- 1 1/2 teaspoon baking powder
- 1/2 teaspoon baking soda
- 1/2 teaspoon salt
- 1/2 teaspoon xanthan gum optional
- 3 eggs
- 1/3 cup coconut oil softened, or butter
- 1/2 cup sweetener Pyure all-purpose
- 2 teaspoons vanilla
- 2 cups zucchini shredded
- 1/2 cup chopped walnuts or pecans

## Directions

1. Combine coconut flour with almond flour, baking powder, cinnamon, baking soda, salt and xanthan gum in a bowl.
2. Whisk eggs with sugar, oil and vanilla in a large bowl.
3. Add the dry mixture into the eggs and mix well.
4. Fold in chopped nuts and shredded zucchini.
5. Spread this mixture over a greased 8x4 silicone bread pan.

6. Place the pan in the slow cooker and cook for about 3 hours on High.

7. Once done, wrap the bread in the foil and serve cool.

**Nutrition**

Calories: 174

Carbs: 13.8g

Fats: 15.7g

Proteins: 5g

Sodium: 247mg

Sugar: 2.4g

# Slow Cooker Cheesy Cauliflower Garlic Bread
**Serves: 8**
**Prep Time: 20mins**

If you haven't yet tried a flourless garlic bread then here is the chance for you, as you can now try this low carb cheesy cauliflower bread. Prepare it out using the mixture of whisked eggs, simple seasoning and minced garlic.   Garnish with chopped basils and enjoy.

## Ingredients
- 12 ounces cauliflower florets (about 1 medium head), finely chopped
- 2 large eggs
- 2 cups shredded mozzarella or Italian cheese blend, divided
- 3 tablespoons coconut flour or other gluten-free flour
- 1/2 teaspoon salt
- 1/2 teaspoon pepper
- 2 cloves garlic, minced
- 1/4 cup chopped fresh basil

## Directions
1. Grease the base of a 6 quart slow cooker with some oil or cooking spray.
2. Mix the chopped cauliflower with eggs, 1 cup shredded cheese, coconut, salt, pepper and gluten free flour in a large bowl.
3. Pour the mixture into the slow cooker and press it firmly with a spoon.
4. Top this layer with garlic and remaining cheese.
5. Cover and cook for 2 to 4 hours on High.
6. Transfer the bread to a serving plate, garnish with basil and slice it to serve.

## Nutrition
Calories: 224
Carbs: 5.6g

Fats: 14.9g
Proteins: 15.6g

Sodium: 249mg
Sugar: 1.5g

# Chicken

## Chicken with Lemon Parsley Butter

**Serves: 10**

**Prep Time: 15 mins**

A nutritious and healthy alternative of traditional roasted chicken, this recipe allows you to cook and steam the chicken slowly which infuses better flavor and aroma. Moreover the butter parsley mixture adds a balance and refreshing taste to the chicken.

### Ingredients

- 1 (5 − 6lbs ) whole roasting chicken, rinsed
- 1 cup water
- 1/2 teaspoon kosher salt
- 1/4 teaspoon ground black pepper
- 1 whole lemon, sliced thinly
- 4 tablespoons butter or ghee
- 2 tablespoons chopped fresh parsley

### Directions

1. Pat dry the chicken and discard all the innards.
2. Season the chicken with salt and pepper then place it at the center of the slow cooker.
3. Pour the water into the cooker just to cover the bottom, add more if needed.
4. Cook the chicken on High for about 3 hours.
5. Add butter, lemon slices and parsley to a saucepan and cook for about 2 minutes until the butter melts.
6. Transfer the cooked chicken to serving dish and pour the lemon sauce over it.

7. Carve and serve warm.

## Nutrition
Calories: 1723

Fats: 116.6g

Sodium: 790mg

Carbs: 0.6g

Proteins: 168.1g

Sugar: 0.2g

# Slow Cooker Paprika Chicken

**Serves: 6**

**Prep Time: 10mins**

With the simplest of the spices readily available in your kitchen the paprika chicken is one easy recipe to cook within few simple steps. All you need is to season the chicken with the desired amount of spices and cook in the slow cooker to blend in, the complete flavor.

## Ingredients

- 1 free range whole chicken
- 1 tablespoon olive oil
- 1 tablespoon dried paprika
- 1 tablespoon curry powder
- 1 teaspoon dried turmeric
- 1 teaspoon salt

## Directions

1. Combine all the spices in a small cup along with oil and salt.
2. Grease the base of your slow cooker and place the chicken in it.
3. Spoon the spice mixture over the chicken and rub it well.
4. Chick on slow for about 6 to 8 hours in the slow cooker.
5. Check if the chicken is al dente by inserting a skewer into its thickest parts.
6. Serve warm and enjoy.

## Nutrition

Calories: 458

Carbs: 1.5g

Fats: 32.9g

Proteins: 37.7g

Sodium: 539mg

Sugar: 0.2g

# Slow Cooker Rotisserie Chicken

**Serves: 4 to 6**

**Prep Time: 15mins**

Rotisserie chicken is one popular recipe which becomes a must have for every special occasion in the house. Now with this slow cooker recipe, you can try it using delicious dried herbs including thyme and rosemary and the juicy flavor of minced garlic. The chicken can be served with warm bread, tortilla or even with rice.

## Ingredients

- 1 organic whole chicken
- 1 tablespoon olive oil
- 1 teaspoon thyme
- 1 teaspoon rosemary
- 1 teaspoon garlic, granulated
- salt and pepper

## Directions

1. Preheat the broiler of your oven.
2. Remove all the giblets from the chicken cavity and place it on the baking tray.
3. Brush the chicken olive oil and top it with spices and herbs.
4. Broil the seasoned chicken in the broiler for about 5 minutes until golden from outside.
5. Meanwhile, roll the aluminum foil pieces into 5 to 6 small balls and place them in the slow cooker.
6. Transfer the chicken from the oven to the cooker and adjust the chicken over the aluminum balls.
7. Cover the lid and cook for 7 to 8 hours on Low setting.

8. Once done, serve warm.

## Nutrition

| | | |
|---|---|---|
| Calories: 265 | Fats: 16.4g | Sodium: 82mg |
| Carbs: 0.4g | Proteins: 27.1g | Sugar: 0g |

# Slow Cooker Chicken Adobo

**Serves: 6**

**Prep Time:  10mins**

The adobo chicken is famous for its enriched tamari flavor with the hints of vinegar. To add a balanced juicy crunch to the chicken it is topped with freshly chopped green onions. Adobo chicken can be best served with cauliflower rice or simple boiled rice.

## Ingredients

- 10-12 chicken drumsticks
- 1 onion, chopped into slices
- 2 tablespoons olive oil
- 10 cloves garlic, crushed
- 1 cup gluten-free tamari soy sauce
- 1/4 cup apple cider vinegar
- 1/4 cup chopped green onion for garnish

## Directions

1. Place the drumsticks in the slow cooker and top them with all the remaining ingredients.
2. Cover the lid and cook for 6 to 8 hours on Low.
3. Once done, top the cooked chicken with green onions.
4. Serve warm.

## Nutrition

Calories: 201

Fats: 9.1g

Sodium: 1317mg

Carbs: 5.1g

Proteins: 24.4g

Sugar: 1g

# Chicken Curry

**Serves: 4**

**Prep Time: 20mins**

This chicken curry recipe is one full package for your dinner table as it is loaded with nutritious coconut milk, delicious spices and juicy onion. With the addition of serrano pepper the chicken gets a new twist to its flavor. Serve warm and fresh for best taste.

## Ingredients

- 1 ½ pounds chicken drumsticks (approx. 5 drumsticks), skin removed
- 1 (13.5 ounce) can organic coconut milk
- 1 onion, finely chopped
- 4 cloves garlic, minced
- 1-inch knob fresh ginger, minced
- 1 Serrano pepper, minced
- 1 tablespoon Garam Masala
- ½ teaspoon cayenne
- ½ teaspoon paprika
- ½ teaspoon turmeric
- salt and pepper, adjust to taste

## Directions

1. Cut the drumsticks around the tendons at the bottom and remove the skin.
2. Add these drumsticks to the slow cooker along with all the remaining ingredients.
3. Cover the lid and cook for 5 to 6 hours on Low setting.
4. Once done, stir well and serve.

## Nutrition

Calories: 528

Carbs: 9.8g

Fats: 32.7g

Proteins: 4926g

Sodium: 156mg

Sugar: 4.6g

# Thai Chicken Curry

**Serves: 4**

**Prep Time: 5mins**

From ages, Thai food has been loved by all for the depth of its flavor and its distinctive aroma. This Thai chicken curry offers you the same with its rich creamy gravy mixed with mouthwatering fish sauce, red curry paste and mixed vegetables. Select the desired combination of the veggies then simply enjoy it with juicy chicken thighs.

## Ingredients

- 1 can coconut milk
- 1/2 cup chicken stock
- 1 lb. boneless, skinless chicken thighs (cut into 1-2 inch pieces)
- 1-2 tablespoons red curry paste
- 1 tablespoon coconut aminos
- 1 tablespoon fish sauce
- 2-3 garlic cloves, minced
- salt and pepper to taste
- red pepper flakes as desired
- 1 bag frozen mixed veggies

## Directions

1. Grease the base of the slow cooker and place the chicken thighs.
2. Mix chicken stock with coconut milk, curry paste, fish sauce, salt, garlic, coconut aminos, pepper and red pepper flakes in a bowl.
3. Pour this mixture over the chicken thighs and cook for 2 hours on High.
4. Add thawed vegetables to the cooker about 30 to 45 minutes before the timer goes off.
5. Mix well and serve warm with spaghetti squash and cauliflower rice.

## Nutrition

Calories: 423          Fats: 24g          Sodium: 774mg

Carbs: 14.8g          Proteins: 36.6g          Sugar: 4.4g

# Slow Cooker Lemongrass and Coconut Chicken Drumsticks

**Serves: 6**

**Prep Time: 45mins**

Lemongrass has very soothing flavor to taste, hence when added to the chicken marinade it gives a defining taste and aroma. The special spices are pureed together to prepare the marinade and then chicken is seasoned with the inviting marinade. Finally the chicken is slow cooked together with the saucy mixture.

## Ingredients

- 10 drumsticks, skin removed
- 1 thick stalk fresh lemongrass, papery outer skins and rough bottom removed, trimmed to the bottom 5 inches
- 4 cloves garlic, minced
- 1 thumb-size piece of ginger
- 1 cup coconut milk
- 2 tablespoons Red Boat fish sauce
- 3 tablespoons coconut aminos
- 1 teaspoon five spice powder
- 1 large onion, thinly sliced
- ¼ cup fresh scallions, chopped
- Kosher salt
- Freshly ground black pepper

## Directions

1. Season the drumsticks with salt and pepper. Keep them aside.
2. Add garlic, ginger, coconut milk, lemongrass, fish sauce, five spice, and coconut aminos to a blender and puree the mixture.

3. Pour the prepared marinade over the seasoned chicken and mix well to coat.
4. Add onions, to the bottom of the slow cooker and top them with chicken along with its marinade.
5. Cook for about 4 to 5 minutes on Low.
6. Once done, serve warm.

## Nutrition

Calories: 477

Fats: 29.6g

Sodium: 771mg

Carbs: 8.8g

Proteins: 41.3g

Sugar: 2.6g

# Green Chile Chicken

**Serves: 6**

**Prep Time: 10mins**

Those who love to eat green chiles, will definitely enjoy this recipe. The chicken is cooked with nothing but green chiles and garlic salt. As there are no other additional spices, it gets the pure taste of garlic and green chiles. For some extra juicy crunch, onions can also be added to the recipe.

## Ingredients

- 6 – 8 boneless skinless chicken thighs, thawed
- 1 can green chiles {4 oz.}
- 2 teaspoons garlic salt
- optional: add in ½ cup diced onions for some extra flavor!

## Directions

1. Add chicken to a greased slow cooker, cover the lid and cook for 6 hours on Low.
2. Once done, transfer the juices from the cooker to a bowl.
3. Add garlic salt and green chiles to the juices and mix well.
4. Pour this mixture over the chicken, cover the lid and cook for another 30 minutes on High.
5. Serve warm with tacos.

## Nutrition

Calories: 164

Carbs: 4g

Fats: 11g

Proteins: 12g

Sodium: 249mg

Sugar: 3g

# Slow Cooker Garlic Butter Chicken with Cream Cheese Sauce

**Serves: 6**

**Prep Time: 10mins**

The special cream cheese sauce makes this recipe a dinner delight for all. First the chicken is slow cooked with rich butter, garlic and salt. Once cooked it is topped with freshly cooked cream cheese sauce which adds a mild and earthy flavor to the juicy chicken.

## Ingredients

For the garlic chicken:

- 2- 2.5 lbs. of chicken breasts
- 1 stick of butter
- 8 garlic cloves, sliced in half to release flavor
- 1.5 teaspoons salt
- Optional -- 1 sliced onion

For the cream cheese sauce:

- 8 oz. of cream cheese
- 1 cup of chicken stock
- salt to taste

## Directions

1. Add the chicken (thawed) to the slow cooker.
2. Add butter, garlic and salt to the chicken and cook on low for about 6 hours.
3. Transfer the chicken onto a serving plate.
4. Add chicken stock to a saucepan along with sat and cream cheese.

5. Cook this mixture over medium low heat until it is combined and creamy.
6. Pour this sauce over the cooked chicken and serve.

**Nutrition**

Calories: 569

Fats: 39.8g

Sodium: 1060mg

Carbs: 4.2g

Proteins: 47.3g

Sugar: 1g

# Jerk chicken

**Serves: 8**

**Prep Time: 10mins**

Season your chicken with simple blend of different peppers, herbs and spices then slow cook to enhance the flavor. When these drumsticks are packed and cooked with the Jerk spice mixture, every bite of it will give a filling flavor. It can be best served with warm tortilla or rice.

## Ingredients

- 5 drumsticks and 5 wings
- 4 teaspoons of salt
- 4 teaspoons of paprika
- 1 teaspoon of cayenne pepper
- 2 teaspoons of onion powder
- 2 teaspoons of thyme
- 2 teaspoons of white pepper
- 2 teaspoons of garlic powder
- 1 teaspoon of black pepper

## Directions

1. Combine all the spices in a bowl and season the washed chicken with this mixture.
2. Place the seasoned chicken in the slow cooker along with all the spices.
3. Cook the chicken on low for 5 to 6 hours until the meat start to fall off from the bones.
4. Serve warm and enjoy.

## Nutrition

Calories: 611          Fats: 32.2g          Sodium: 2678mg
Carbs: 2.5g            Proteins: 72.5g      Sugar: 0.5g

# Pork

## Slow-Cooked Keto Pork Roast with Creamy Gravy

**Serves: 6**

**Prep Time: 5 mins**

For a slow cooked pork roast, the meat is generously seasoned with a blend of delicious spices and cooked for hours to infuse a perfect flavor. Further it is roasted in the oven to add more crisp and color. Serve with creamy rich gravy for best taste.

### Ingredients

- 2 lbs. pork shoulder or pork roast
- ½ tablespoon salt
- 1 bay leaf
- 5 black peppercorns
- 2½ cups water
- 2 teaspoons dried thyme or dried rosemary
- 2 garlic cloves
- 1½ oz. fresh ginger
- 1 tablespoon olive oil or coconut oil
- 1 tablespoon paprika powder
- ½ teaspoon ground black pepper

Creamy gravy:
- 1½ cups heavy whipping cream
- juices from the roast

### Directions

1. Preheat your slow cooker on low.
2. Season the meat with salt and place it in the slow cooker.

3. Add 1 cup water to the meat along with thyme, peppercorns and bay.
4. Cover and cook for about 8 hours on low setting or for 4 hours in high.
5. Once done, reserve the cooking liquid aside and keep the meat aside.
6. Preheat your oven to 450°F (220°C).
7. Mix garlic, ginger, oil, peppers and herbs in a bowl and season the pork with this mixture.
8. Place the meat in a well-greased baking dish and bake for about 10 to 15 minutes.
9. Mix cream with cooking liquid to prepare the gravy.
10. Serve warm with creamy gravy.

## Nutrition

Calories: 938

Fats: 77.2g

Sodium: 784g

Carbs: 12.8g

Proteins: 40.1g

Sugar: 1.1g

# Slow Cooker Pulled Pork Recipe

## Serves: 6

## Prep Time: 10mins

You may have tried different versions of pulled pork but this bbq sauce glazed pork is absolutely delicious. Firstly the meat is cooked with its own spices in the slow cooker, to enhance its natural flavor then a special bbq sauce is prepared to mix with shredded meat. The mixture can be used as sandwich or tacos filling or can also be served with rice or bread.

## Ingredients

For the pulled pork:

- 3lb boneless pork shoulder (aka. Boston Butt)
- 1 teaspoon onion powder
- 1 teaspoon garlic powder
- 1 teaspoon kosher salt
- 1/2 teaspoons black pepper
- 1/2 teaspoons paprika
- 1/2 teaspoons ground allspice
- 1/2 teaspoons celery salt
- 1/8 teaspoons ground cloves
- 1/2 teaspoons mustard powder
- 1/2 cup water

For The Bbq Sauce:

- 1/2 teaspoons ground allspice
- 1/4 cup prepared yellow mustard
- 2 teaspoons hot sauce
- 3 tablespoons apple cider vinegar
- 3 tablespoons low sugar ketchup

- 4 tablespoons granulated sugar substitute
- 1/2 teaspoons xanthan gum

## Directions

1. Mix salt with onion powder, paprika, pepper, garlic powder, celery salt, allspice, mustard powder and cloves in a small bowl.
2. Season the pork with the spice mixture and place it in the slow cooker.
3. Add water to the pork and cover the lid. Cook for 4 hours on high until the meat is al dente.
4. Shred the cooked meat using two forks and keep it aside.
5. Keep the cooking liquid and skim off the excess fats and discard.
6. Mix the cooking liquid with all the sauce ingredients in the slow cooker.
7. Cover the lid and cook for 10 minutes on high.
8. Return the pork shreds to the cooker and mix well with the sauce.
9. Serve warm.

## Nutrition

Calories: 350        Fats: 8.5g        Sodium: 900mg
Carbs: 8.4g          Proteins: 60.4g   Sugar: 2.4g

# Low Carb Pork Chops with Spice Rub

**Serves: 8**

**Prep Time: 15mins**

Experience these slow cooked pork chops, which are cooked with the unique blend of chives, fennel seeds and dried herbs. For better taste, the seasoned chops can also be marinated overnight in the refrigerator. Once refrigerated, let them sit at room temperature for 15 minutes before cooking.

## Ingredients

- 1 tablespoon rosemary dried
- 1 tablespoon thyme dried
- 1 tablespoon curry powder dried
- 1 tablespoon chives chopped, fresh
- 1 tablespoon fennel seeds
- 1 tablespoon ground cumin
- 1 teaspoon salt
- 4 tablespoons olive oil
- 2 pounds pork chops

## Directions

1. Mix salt, fennel seeds, thyme, rosemary, chives. Cumin, 2 tablespoons olive oil and salt in a large bowl.
2. Season the pork chops with the prepared mixture and mix well.
3. Grease the slow cooker with remaining oil and place the seasoned chops in the cooker.
4. Cover the lid and cook for 6 hours on medium setting.

## Nutrition

Calories: 433

Carbs: 1.7g

Fats: 35.7g

Proteins: 25.9g

Sodium: 373mg

Sugar: 0.1g

# Pork Carnitas

**Serves: 16**

**Prep Time:   10mins**

Here is another, festive dinner delight for your family. Pork carnitas is one easy and effortless dish to prepare. First the pork is rubbed with spices then cooked over a layer of onion and garlic. This gives the meat a tempting aroma of onion and garlic. Serve warm with steaming rice or sautéed vegetables.

## Ingredients
- 8 lb. boston pork butt
- 2 tablespoons bacon grease
- 1 large onion
- 2 tablespoons cumin
- 2 tablespoons thyme
- 2 tablespoons chili powder
- 1 tablespoon salt
- 1 tablespoon pepper
- 4 tablespoons minced garlic
- 1 cup water

## Directions
1. Grease the slow cooker with bacon fats.
2. Add onions to the cooker then top them with garlic.
3. Remove the fats from the meat and cut it in crisscross pattern.
4. Season the meat with all the spice and rub it well generously.
5. Sprinkle the excess spices over the onion and garlic.
6. Add the meat to the cooker and top it with 1 cup of water.
7. Cover the lid and cook on high for about 8 hours.
8. Once done, serve warm.

## Nutrition
Calories: 609          Fats: 45g          Sodium: 655mg
Carbs: 5g              Proteins: 54g      Sugar: 0.2g

# Easy slow cooker pork steaks recipe

**Serves: 4**

**Prep Time: 20mins**

Try these luscious pork steaks with the aroma of pork rub, celtic salt and freshly cracked pepper. Simply season the steaks with the spices and slow cook for some hours and voila, the steaming steaks are ready to be served.

## Ingredients

- 4 pork steaks
- 2 tablespoons pork rub
- 1 teaspoon celtic sea salt
- 1 teaspoon fresh cracked pepper

## Directions

1. Pat dry the pork steaks and season them with all the spices.
2. Place the steaks in the slow cooker and cover the lid.
3. Cook on high for about 4 to 6 hours.
4. Once the timer goes off, check the tenderness of the meat with a fork.
5. Serve with vegetables, rice or salad.

## Nutrition

Calories: 450

Carbs: 1.8g

Fats: 28.1g

Proteins: 43.3g

Sodium: 710mg

Sugar: 0.8g

# Pork Roast

**Serves: 4**
**Prep Time: 5mins**

There is no better combination than pork with bacon. And when these two are paired with delicious bbq sauce, the flavor gets a new twist and tempting aroma. After slow cooking, the pork roast is broiled to achieve a nice brown color and some crisp.

## Ingredients

- 2.5 pound pork loin roast
- 1.5 cups sugar free bbq sauce
- 5 slices thick cut bacon

## Directions

1. Add the pork loin to the slow cooker and top it with half of the bbq sauce.
2. Place the bacon slices over it and pour the remaining bbq sauce.
3. Cover the lid and cook on Low setting for about 4 hours.
4. Meanwhile, preheat the broiler 15 minutes before the slow cooker's timer goes off.
5. Roast the cooked loin along with its sauce in the broiler for about 5 minutes.
6. Serve warm and enjoy.

## Nutrition

Calories: 698          Fats: 33.6g          Sodium: 1047mg
Carbs: 6g              Proteins: 86.1g      Sugar: 0g

# Slow Cooker Ranch Pork Chops

**Serves: 6**

**Prep Time: 45mins**

With the refreshing ranch dressing sauce mixed with mushrooms and cream of chicken soup, the pork loins taste amazingly delicious. Serve it with the healthy mix of mashed cauliflower or with fresh or sautéed vegetables for a complete meal.

## Ingredients

- 2 lbs. of Pork Loin, thawed
- 2 cans Cream of Chicken Soup
- 2 cups Water
- 1 Packet Ranch Dressing Mix
- 1 8oz Container of Sliced Mushrooms (optional)

## Directions

1. Mix cream of chicken soup, ranch dressing, and 2 cups of water in a mixing bowl.
2. Fold in mushrooms and mix well to coat.
3. Slice the pork loins into 6 slices then place them in the slow cooker.
4. Top the pork with prepared sauce and cover the lid.
5. Cook for about 8 hours on low.
6. Once done, serve with sautéed vegetables or mashed cauliflower.

## Nutrition

Calories: 488

Carbs: 11.4g

Fats: 26.9g

Proteins: 45.8g

Sodium: 1334mg

Sugar: 2.6g

# Slow Cooked Pork Roast with Cheese

**Serves: 6**

**Prep Time: 20mins**

Serve the pork roast with rich cheesy cream gravy. First the roast is slow cooked with mushrooms, celery and all the juicy vegetables then mixed with the blend of cream, cheese, butter and Glucomannan powder.

## Ingredients

- 1 large pork roast - bone-in or boneless is fine
- 1 1/2 cups chicken stock
- 1 cup diced onion
- 1/2 cup finely diced mushrooms
- 3-4 celery stalks, chopped
- 1/4 cup dried parsley
- 1/2 stick butter
- 2 teaspoons salt
- 1 teaspoon garlic powder
- 1 teaspoon black pepper

For the Gravy:
- 1 cup heavy cream
- 4 ounces cream cheese, cubed
- 1/2 stick butter
- 1/2-1 teaspoon Glucomannan powder
- 1 1/2-2 cups cooking liquid from roast

## Directions

1. Add pork roast to the slow cooker along with mushrooms, onions and celery.

2. Pour chicken broth into the cooker and add seasoning with 1/2 stick butter.
3. Cover the lid and cook on low for about 6 to 8 hours.
4. Once cooked, remove the roast from the cooker and keep it aside. Cover to keep it warm.
5. Prepare gravy by adding 4 oz. cream cheese. 1/2 stick butter and 1 cup heavy cream to a saucepan.
6. Heat this mixture over medium high heat and whisk well until butter melts to form a smooth liquid.
7. Add 1/2 teaspoon Glucomannan powder which stirring then bring the mixture to a boil.
8. Cook for 2 minutes, mix well then reduce the heat to cooker for another 5 minutes.
9. Cook until the gravy thicken, add more Glucomannan if needed.
10. Adjust the seasoning with salt and pepper then pour the gravy over the cooked roast.
11. Serve warm.

**Nutrition**

Calories: 463      Fats: 42.1g      Sodium: 1125mg

Carbs: 4.4g      Proteins: 17.9g      Sugar: 1.4g

# Balsamic Pork Roast

**Serves: 6**

**Prep Time: 10mins**

The balsamic glazed pork shoulders are best for dinner table, as they are prepared with a mild blend of sweet and sour. Mixed with honey and Worcestershire sauce the pork can be best served with rice or warm tortilla.

## Ingredients

- 2 pound boneless pork shoulder roast (sirloin roast)
- kosher salt, to taste
- 1/2 teaspoons garlic powder
- ½ teaspoon red pepper flakes
- 1/3 cup chicken or vegetable broth
- 1/3 cup balsamic vinegar
- 1 tablespoon Worcestershire sauce
- 1 tablespoon honey

## Directions

1. Season the meat with garlic powder, red pepper flakes and salt.
2. Place the seasoned pork into the slow cooker.
3. Mix vinegar, broth and Worcestershire sauce in a small bowl and pour it over the pork.
4. Top the meat with honey then cook for 4 hours on high setting.
5. Once done, transfer the pork to the serving plate and shred it using a fork.
6. Top the meat with warm sauce and serve.

## Nutrition

Calories: 417     Fats: 31.1g     Sodium: 161mg
Carbs: 3.8g       Proteins: 27.7g     Sugar: 3.5g

# Slow Cooker Chipotle Pork

## Serves: 8 to 10
## Prep Time: 20mins

Chipotle peppers are known for their good spice and mild tangy taste. Along with other dried herbs, tomatoes and green chiles, the chipotle peppers gives a perfect balance to the pork shoulders. Garnish with fresh cilantro and serve warm.

## Ingredients
- 6 lbs. pork shoulder
- 4 garlic cloves sliced thin
- 2 teaspoons salt
- 2 teaspoons garlic powder
- 2 teaspoons oregano
- 2 tablespoons cumin
- 4 teaspoons ground coriander
- 4 teaspoons chili powder
- 1/2 teaspoon black pepper
- 1/2 teaspoon onion powder
- 1 tablespoon of olive oil
- 4 tablespoons apple cider vinegar
- 2 cups peppers sliced
- 1 onion sliced
- 1 7 oz. can of chipotle peppers
- 1 14.5 oz. can diced tomatoes
- 1 4 oz. can of green chiles

## Directions
1. Carve few slits in the pork roast and stuff it with garlic generously.
2. Mix all the dry spices in a bowl and rub the mixture over the pork.

3. Add oil to a large skillet and sea the roast on medium high heat for about 4 minutes per side.
4. Reduce the heat to medium then add tomatoes, vinegar, chipotles and chiles to the skillet.
5. Stir cook for about 5 minutes then transfer the mixture to the slow cooker along with peppers and onions.
6. Mix well then top this mixture with seared roast. Cook for about 6 to 8 hours on medium.
7. When the timer goes off, remove the roast from the cooker and pull its meat to shred.
8. Return the shreds to the cooker and mix well.
9. Serve warm with tacos or rice.

**Nutrition**

Calories: 861

Fats: 61.6g

Sodium: 741mg

Carbs: 7.6g

Proteins: 66g

Sugar: 3.3g

# Beef

## Keto Slow-Cooker Beef & Broccoli

**Serves: 6**

**Prep Time: 10 mins**

There is no better way to get a good taste of broccoli than to pair it with slow cooked juicy beef.   The beef steaks are first cooked with a mix of tangy and sweet blend of spices. The broccoli and red bell are added later to keep their juicy crunch fresh for every bite.

### Ingredients

- 2 lbs. flank steak, slice into 2" chunks
- 2/3 cup liquid aminos
- 1 cup beef broth
- 3 tablespoons your sweetener of choice
- 1 teaspoon freshly grated ginger
- 3 garlic cloves, minced
- 1/4 - 1/2 teaspoons red pepper flakes
- 1/2 teaspoons salt
- 1 head broccoli, chopped
- 1 red bell pepper, chopped
- 1 teaspoon sesame seeds (garnish)

### Directions

1. Add steak, aminos, beef broth, ginger, sweetener, red pepper flakes and salt to the slow cooker.
2. Cook for 5 to 6 hours on low setting.
3. Once done, add broccoli and red bell to the steaks. Cook for another 1 hour.
4. Sprinkle with sesame seeds and serve.

### Nutrition

Calories: 320

Carbs: 4.6g

Fats: 13.2g

Proteins: 46.4g

Sodium: 2118mg

Sugar: 2.4g

# Low Carb Beef Stroganoff

**Serves: 6**

**Prep Time: 5 mins**

Beef Stroganoff is one popular meal which is cooked with mushrooms and rich tomato paste. And this stroganoff is supremely delicious as the beef and all the ingredients are slow cooked together for hours. When served with sour cream or cream cheese, it tastes more scrumptious than ever.

## Ingredients

- 1 brown onion sliced and quartered
- 2 cloves garlic crushed
- 2 slices streaky bacon diced
- 1 lb. beef, stewing steak cubed
- 1 teaspoon smoked paprika
- 3 tablespoons tomato paste
- 1 cup beef stock
- ½ cup mushrooms quartered

## Directions

1. Add all the ingredients to the slow cooker and mix well.
2. Cover and cook on low for 6 to 8 hours or on High for 4 to 6 hours.
3. Serve warm with cream cheese or sour cream.

## Nutrition

Calories: 260

Fats: 14.2g

Sodium: 865mg

Carbs: 6g

Proteins: 26.5g

Sugar: 3.2g

# Slow Cooker Malaysian Beef Curry

**Serves: 6**

**Prep Time: 5 mins**

There are not many Malaysian recipes that most of us know well, but if you want to try something different and exotic then here is a Malaysian beef curry recipe. Besides good amount of beef, there is a rich coconut cream and special Chinese five spice, which will make your mouth water instantly.

## Ingredients

- 1 ½ lbs. beef suitable for stewing/casserole cut into large pieces
- ½ cup coconut cream
- 1 red onion quartered
- 1 teaspoon ground cardamom
- 1 teaspoon Chinese five spice
- 1/2 teaspoons chilli powder
- 1 teaspoon ground cinnamon
- 2 teaspoons coriander/cilantro ground
- 1 teaspoon ground cumin
- 1 teaspoon turmeric
- 4 cloves whole
- large handful of leafy greens

## Directions

1. Add coconut cream along with spices to the slow cooker and mix well.
2. Stir in beef and onion then cook for 8 to 10 hours on Low or 4 to 6 hours on High.
3. Once done, add the leafy greens to the beef and let it stay for 5 minutes then mix gently.

4. Serve warm.

**Nutrients**

Calories: 256

Fats: 14.1g

Sodium: 745mg

Carbs: 2g

Proteins: 29.1g

Sugar: 1.4g

# Picadillo

**Serves: 6**

**Prep Time: 10mins**

Picadillo is one flavorsome Cuban dish which is made out of delicious green olives, juicy bell peppers, tomatoes and a balance amount of spices. Try this slow cooker picadillo recipe and surprise your family at the special weeknight dinners or any other festive occasion of the year.

## Ingredients

- 2 1/2 lbs. 93% lean ground beef
- 1 cup minced onion
- 1 cup diced red bell peppers
- 3 cloves garlic, minced
- 1/4 cup minced cilantro
- 1 small tomato, diced
- 8 oz. can tomato sauce
- 1/4 cup alcaparrado (manzanilla olives, pimientos, capers) or green olives
- 1 1/2 teaspoons ground cumin
- 1/4 teaspoons garlic powder
- 2 bay leaves
- kosher salt and fresh pepper, to taste

## Directions

1. Sear the meat in a large skillet over medium high heat while sprinkling salt and pepper over it.
2. Cook until meat is brown then add garlic, onion and bell peppers to the skillet. Sauté for 3 to 4 minutes.

3. Transfer this mixture to the slow cooker and add cilantro, tomato, water, tomato sauce and alcaparrado.
4. Add all the remaining ingredients and slow cook on low for 6 to 8 hours or on high for about 3 to 4 hours.
5. Once done, discard the bay leaves and serve warm with brown rice.

**Nutrition**

Calories: 207

Fats: 8.5g

Sodium: 655mg

Carbs: 5g

Proteins: 28g

Sugar: 3g

# Garlic Beef Stew with Olives, Capers and Tomatoes

## Serves: 6

## Prep Time: 20mins

Create an inspiring, sweet and luscious garlic beef stew with a generous amount of garlic, tomatoes, capers and olives. The chuck roast beef is first seared than cooked with all the spices and vegetables in the slow cooker for hours.

## Ingredients

- 2-3 lb. beef chuck roast, cut into pieces about 1 inch (I used 2 1/2 cups beef cubes)
- 1-2 tablespoons olive oil (for browning beef)
- 1 can reduced-sodium beef broth (or use 1 1/2 cups homemade beef stock)
- 1 cup garlic cloves, peeled and cut into lengthwise slivers
- 1 cup Kalamata Olives, cut in half lengthwise
- 2 tablespoons capers, rinsed
- 3 bay leaves
- 1 teaspoon dried Greek oregano
- 1 can (14.5 oz.) diced tomatoes with juice
- 1 small can (8 oz.) tomato sauce
- 2 tablespoons tomato paste
- 3 tablespoons red wine vinegar
- fresh ground black pepper to taste

## Directions

1. Heat oil in a skillet over medium high heat.
2. Add beef cubes and cook until brown from all the sides.
3. Transfer the beef cubes to the slow cooker.

4. Pour the beef broth into the skillet and let it simmer until it is reduced to 3/4 cup.
5. Transfer the broth to the cooker and add olives, garlic, bay leaves, oregano, capers, juice, tomato paste, sauce, red wine, pepper and tomatoes.
6. Cook on high for 4 hours.
7. Serve warm.

**Nutrition**

Calories: 153

Fats: 6g

Sodium: 44mg

Carbs: 3g

Proteins: 19g

Sugar: 1.3g

# Slow Cooker Kickin' Chili

## Serves: 5

## Prep Time: 30mins

Have chili filled gluten free beef treat for an inviting meal. The beef is stewed together with tangy Mexican seasoning and tomatoes. Further a flavorsome mix of Worcestershire sauce and jalapenos slices is added to enhance the flavor.

## Ingredients

- 2 1/2 lbs. ground beef
- 1 medium red onion, chopped and divided
- 4 tablespoons minced garlic
- 3 large ribs of celery, diced
- ¼ cup pickled jalapeno slices
- 6 oz. can tomato paste
- 14.5 oz. can tomatoes and green chilies
- 14.5 oz. can stewed tomatoes with Mexican seasoning
- 2 tablespoons Worcestershire sauce or Coconut Aminos
- 4 tablespoons chili powder
- 2 tablespoons cumin, mounded
- 2 teaspoons sea salt
- 1/2 teaspoons cayenne
- 1 teaspoon garlic powder
- 1 teaspoon onion powder
- 1 teaspoon oregano
- 1 teaspoon black pepper
- 1 bay leaf

## Directions

1. Add beef with half of onions, 2 tablespoons, garlic, pepper and salt to a large and sauté until golden brown.
2. Drain the excess fats and transfer the beef mixture to the slow cooker.
3. Add all the remaining ingredients to the slow cooker and mix well.
4. Cook on low for about 6 to 8 hours.

## Nutrients

Calories: 137

Carbs: 4.7g

Fats: 15g

Proteins: 16g

Sodium: 249mg

Sugar: 1.3g

# Green Chile Shredded Beef Cabbage Bowl with Avocado Salsa

**Serves: 6**

**Prep Time: 20 mins**

Prepare to get a perfect treat for your special dinner with the spicy beef shreds, juicy cabbage salad and tempting avocado salsa. The chuck roast when cooked with taco seasoning and green chiles becomes irresistible and that avocado salsa is simply crowd pleasing.

## Ingredients

for Slow Cooker Beef:

- 2 lb. beef chuck roast, well-trimmed and cut into thick strips
- 1 tablespoon kalyn's taco seasoning
- 2-3 teaspoons olive oil
- 2 cans (4 oz. can) diced green chiles with juice
- For Cabbage Slaw and Dressing:
- 1 small head green cabbage
- 1/2 small head red cabbage
- 1/2 cup thinly sliced green onion
- 6 tablespoons mayo or light mayo
- 4 teaspoons fresh squeezed lime juice
- 2 teaspoons green tabasco sauce

For the Avocado Salsa:

- 2 large avocados, diced
- 1 medium Poblano (Passilla) pepper, diced very small
- 1 tablespoon fresh-squeezed lime juice
- 1 tablespoon extra-virgin olive oil
- 1/2 cup finely chopped cilantro

## Directions

1. Remove all the fats from the beef and cut it into thick strips.
2. Season the meat with taco seasonings and sear the season beef in heated oil until brown from all the sides.
3. Once seared transfer the beef to the slow cooker and green chiles along with their juices.
4. Cook for about 3 to 4 hours on high setting.
5. Transfer the beef to the cutting board with a slotted spoon and shred the meat using two forks.
6. Return the shred to the slow cooker and cover the lid to keep it warm.
7. Mix mayo with green tabasco and lime juice. Add green onions and cabbage to the mixture and toss well.
8. Mix avocado with lime juice, cilantro and Poblano Chile in a bowl.
9. Serve the beef with avocado mix and cabbage salad.

## Nutrition

Calories: 818

Fats: 64g

Sodium: 454mg

Carbs: 15.5g

Proteins: 42.2g

Sugar: 4.2g

# Chipotle Barbacoa Recipe

**Serves: 9**

**Prep Time: 10mins**

This copycat Barbacoa recipe sounds even more scrumptious due to the blend of apple cider vinegar with chipotle chiles, lime juice and other earthy spices. The comforting beef recipe take less of your kitchen time, as the ingredients are simply blended and slow cooked without taking much of your efforts.

## Ingredients

- 3 lb. Beef brisket or chuck roast
- 1/2 cup Beef broth
- 2 medium Chipotle chiles in adobo
- 5 cloves Garlic
- 2 tablespoons Apple cider vinegar
- 2 tablespoons Lime juice
- 1 tablespoon dried oregano
- 2 teaspoons Cumin
- 2 teaspoons Sea salt
- 1 teaspoon Black pepper
- 1/2 teaspoons Ground cloves
- 2 whole Bay leaf

## Direction

1. Add all the ingredients to a blender except beef and bay leaves. Blend until it forms a smooth paste.
2. Place the beef chunks into the slow cooker and top them with spice mixture and bay leaves.
3. Cook for about to 6 hours on high and 8 to 10 hours on low setting.

4. Once cooked, discard the bay leaves and remove the beef chunks from the cooker.
5. Shred the meat using two forks and return it to the cooker, mix well and cover the lid for 5 to 10 minutes.
6. Serve warm and enjoy.

**Nutrition**

Calories: 242

Fats: 11g

Sodium: 854mg

Carbs: 1g

Proteins: 32g

Sugar: 0.3g

# Low-Carb Southwestern Pot Roast in the Slow Cooker

**Serves: 8**

**Prep Time: 10mins**

This pot roast is simple a salsa soaked beef meat which is seared and slow cooked for better taste and aroma. The salsa is added at different stages of cooking so that it flavor would slowly penetrate deep into the boneless beef meat.

## Ingredients

- 3 lb. boneless chuck roast, trimmed of visible fat
- 1 can (14 oz.) reduced sodium beef broth
- 1 1/4 cup your favorite salsa
- 1-2 teaspoons olive oil for browning meat

## Directions

1. Cook beef broth in a saucepan until it is reduced to half cup. Skim off all the surface fats.
2. Heat oil in a large skillet and brown the beef from all the sides over medium heat.
3. Transfer the meat to the slow cooker and top it with beef broth and 1 cup salsa.
4. Cover the lid and cook on high for 1 hour or 3 to 4 hours on low setting.
5. Remove the fats from the sauce and stir in remaining salsa. Cook more until the sauce is reduced to about 1 cup.
6. Mix well and serve warm.

## Nutrition

Calories: 584

Carbs: 2.6g

Fats: 41.3g

Proteins: 47.9g

Sodium: 508mg

Sugar: 1.2g

# Low Carb Slow Cooker Chinese Five-Spice Beef

**Serves: 6**

**Prep Time: 10mins**

A nice blend of beef with juicy vegetables and greens is what this recipe offers. It is full of snow peas, bell pepper, savory mushrooms, green onions and plenty of other easily available veggies. The meat is first seared then cooked with a delicious gravy which can be best served with steaming rice or over a bowl of your favorite pasta.

## Ingredients

- 2 pounds stew beef
- Sea salt and ground black pepper
- 2 tablespoons olive oil
- 1 cup beef stock
- 1/2 cup cooking sherry
- 1/4 cup coconut aminos or gluten free soy sauce
- 2 tablespoons unseasoned rice wine vinegar
- 2 red bell peppers, seeded and sliced
- 8 ounces cremini mushrooms, quartered
- 2 large shallots, thinly sliced
- 3 cloves garlic, minced
- 1 (2-inch) piece fresh ginger, grated
- 1 tablespoon plus 1 teaspoon Chinese five-spice powder
- 1 teaspoon red pepper flakes
- 2 cups snow peas
- 2 green onions, sliced on the bias, for garnish
- 2 tablespoons toasted sesame seeds, for garnish

## Directions

1. Season the stew beef with pepper and salt. Sear it in a skillet over medium heat until brown from all the side.
2. Transfer the meat to the slow cooker along with its juices.
3. Add all the remaining ingredients to the cooker except peas, sesame seeds and green onions.
4. Cover the lid and cook for 6 hours on medium setting.
5. When the timer goes off stir in snow peas and cook for 1 hour.
6. Garnish with sesame seeds and green onions then serve warm.

**Nutrition**

Calories: 337
Carbs: 10.8g

Fats: 15.7g
Proteins: 37.6g

Sodium: 138mg
Sugar: 4.8g

# Soups

## Cabbage Soup Recipe

**Serves: 10**

**Prep Time: 5 mins**

Enriched with the protein filled beef and fibers, this soup is one warming delight for the dinner table. As the beef ground is first seared along with the juicy onion, it adds an extra crisp and balanced crunch to the tomato loaded cabbage soup. For best taste, serve with warm bread.

### Ingredients
- 2 pounds Ground Beef 90% lean
- 1/4 onion large, diced
- 1 clove garlic minced
- 1 teaspoon cumin ground
- 1 head cabbage large, chopped
- 4 cubes bouillon
- 10 oz. Rotel Diced Tomatoes & Green Chilies 1 can
- 4 cups water
- Salt and pepper to taste

### Directions
1. Sauté ground beef over medium heat in a skillet then add onion and cook for about 2 minutes.
2. Transfer this mixture to the slow cooker.
3. Add cabbage, garlic, cumin, tomatoes, bouillon cubes, water and green chilies.
4. Slow cook for about 2 to 3 hours over high heat.
5. Mix well and serve warm.

### Nutrition
Calories: 236          Fats: 11.1g          Sodium: 457mg
Carbs: 5.9g            Proteins: 27.2g      Sugar: 3.4g

# Homemade Thai Chicken Soup

**Serves: 10**

**Prep Time: 10mins**

The homemade Thai chicken soup is absolutely effortless, as it requires some few basic ingredients from your kitchen shelf. Add them together and let your slow cooker take care of the rest. All these ingredients when cooked slowly with lemon grass stalks, the soup gets an inspiring new aroma and flavor.

## Ingredients

- 1 whole chicken, cut into small pieces
- 1 stalk of lemongrass, cut into large chunks
- 20 fresh basil leaves (10 for the slow cooker, and 10 for garnish)
- 5 thick slices of fresh ginger
- 1 lime
- 1 Tablespoon salt
- Additional salt to taste

## Directions

1. Add chicken, 10 basil leaves, lemongrass, salt and ginger to the slow cooker.
2. Fill the cooker with water and cook on low for about 8 to 10 hours.
3. Once done, transfer the soup to the serving bowl and adjust the seasoning with salt and lime juice.
4. Garnish it with basil leaves.
5. Serve warm.

## Nutrition

Calories: 99

Carbs: 7.7g

Fats: 12g

Proteins: 11.3g

Sodium: 1778mg

Sugar: 0.4g

# Slow Cooker Chicken Bacon Chowder

**Serves: 8**

**Prep Time: 15mins**

Chowders are loved for their rich and creamy taste and texture, whereas this chicken bacon chowder twice more delicious than any other as it is packed with chopped leek, celery and mushrooms. Cream together with cheese makes it healthy and nutritious for all.

## Ingredients

- 4 cloves garlic, minced
- 1 shallot, finely chopped
- 1 small leek, cleaned, trimmed and sliced
- 2 ribs celery, diced
- 6 oz. cremini mushrooms, sliced
- 1 medium sweet onion, thinly sliced
- 4 tablespoons butter, divided
- 2 cups chicken stock, divided
- 1 lb. chicken breasts
- 8 oz. cream cheese
- 1 cup heavy cream
- 1 lb. bacon, cooked crisp and crumbled
- 1 teaspoon sea salt
- 1 teaspoon black pepper
- 1 teaspoon garlic powder
- 1 teaspoon dried thyme

## Directions

1. Add garlic, leek, shallot, mushrooms, celery, onions, 1 cup chicken stock, 2 tablespoons Butter, sea salt and black pepper to the slow cooker.

2. Cover the lid and slow cook for about 1 hour on Low heat.
3. Meanwhile, stir fry the chicken with 2 tablespoons butter in a large skillet over medium high heat.
4. Cook the chicken for about 5 minutes from both the sides.
5. Transfer the chicken to a plate and keep it aside.
6. Deglaze the skillet with remaining chicken stock and scrape off the chicken bits from the base.
7. Transfer this chicken stock to the slow cooker.
8. Stir in cream cheese, heavy cream, and thyme and garlic powder and mix well.
9. Dice the chicken into cubes and transfer it to the cooker along with bacon.
10. Cook for about 6 to 8 hours.
11. Once done, serve immediately.

## Nutrition

Calories: 646

Fats: 49.4g

Sodium: 1927mg

Carbs: 8g

Proteins: 41.3g

Sugar: 1.9g

# Keto Chicken Cordon Bleu Soup

**Serves: 8**

**Prep Time:   10mins**

Unlike other soups, this one is made out diced ham which is paired with chicken. Such blend of proteins is not only unique in flavor but also rich in content. Along with basic spices like salt and pepper, dried tarragon is also added to give a new twist to its flavor.

## Ingredients

- 6 cups chicken stock
- 12 ounces diced ham
- 5 ounces mushrooms, chopped
- 4 ounces onion, diced
- 2 teaspoons dried tarragon
- 1 teaspoon sea salt, more to taste
- 1 teaspoon black pepper
- 1 pound chicken breast, cubed
- 4 cloves garlic, minced
- 3 tablespoons salted butter
- 1 1/2 cups heavy cream
- 1/2 cup sour cream
- 1/2 cup grated Parmesan cheese
- 4 ounces Swiss cheese

## Directions

1. Add ham, chicken stock, onion, tarragon, mushrooms, salt and pepper to the slow cooker.
2. Cover the lid and set the cooker on Low for 6 hours.
3. Meanwhile sear the chicken with butter in a skillet along with garlic until it is brown and crispy.

4. Transfer the cooked chicken to the cooker along with the drippings.
5. Add Parmesan cheese, heavy cream, sour cream and swish cheese to the cooker.
6. Cover the lid and cook for 6 hours.
7. When the timer goes off, mix well and serve warm.

**Nutrition**

Calories: 535

Carbs: 8.8g

Fats: 37.2g

Proteins: 43.3g

Sodium: 1986mg

Sugar: 1.7g

# No Noodle Chicken Soup

## Serves: 10

## Prep Time: 10mins

The no noodle chicken soup is made out of savory vegetables which are slow cooked together with the chicken bones for hours. As the vegetables can be selected as per the desired taste, so opt the ones which are full of fibers and essential vitamins to make this soup even healthier.

## Ingredients

- 1 whole chicken
- 2 bunches celery, chopped into 4 inch pieces
- 3 tablespoons salt
- 1 teaspoon black pepper
- 6 cups water
- 4 cups mixed frozen vegetables

## Directions

1. Add celery to the base of the slow cooker and top it with chicken.
2. Drizzle salt and pepper over the chicken then cover the lid and cook for 8 to 10 hours.
3. Once the timer goes off, remove the chicken from the cooker and pull the meat from the bones.
4. Shred and preserve the meat in the refrigerate using a sealed bag.
5. Return the bones to the slow cooker and add water then cook for 6 to 8 hours.
6. Strain the soup, discard all the solids then return the stock to the cooker.

7. Add celery, vegetables, shredded chicken, salt and pepper to the stock and cook on High until veggies are al dente.
8. When done, serve warm.

**Nutrition**

| | | |
|---|---|---|
| Calories: 865 | Fats: 56.1g | Sodium: 2436mg |
| Carbs: 5.1g | Proteins: 85.1g | Sugar: 1.3g |

# White Chicken Chili Soup

## Serves: 6 to 8

## Prep Time: 5mins

The white chicken chili soup is famous for the combination of the spices it incorporates, as there is jalapeno, oregano, coriander and cumin along with many others on the list. The given measurements can be changed as per the desired taste and hotness, reduce the pepper if you want to avoid extra tanginess.

## Ingredients

- 2 pounds boneless, skinless chicken breasts
- 2 onions, diced
- 4 stalks celery, diced
- 1-2 jalapeño pepper, minced
- 10 cloves garlic, minced
- 1 tablespoon chili powder
- 1 tablespoon salt, adjust to taste
- 1 teaspoon cumin
- 1 teaspoon coriander powder
- 1 teaspoon oregano
- ½ teaspoon freshly crushed black pepper, adjust to taste
- 4 cups chicken broth
- Serve with cilantro, hot sauce, cheese if desired

## Directions

1. Add all the ingredients to the slow cooker except for corn and cannellini beans.
2. Cover the lid and cook the mixture for about 4 hours on High setting.
3. Remove the lid about 30 minutes before the timer goes off.

4. Remove the chicken from the cooker and shred it using a fork.

5. Add the chicken shreds, corn and cannellini to the cooker.

6. Let it cook for remaining 30 minutes then mix well.

7. Serve warm.

## Nutrients

| | | |
|---|---|---|
| Calories: 344 | Fats: 12.5g | Sodium: 1826mg |
| Carbs: 7.3g | Proteins: 48.1g | Sugar: 2.4g |

# Creamy Lemon Chicken Kale Soup

## Serves: 6

## Prep Time: 15mins

The green kale soup is cooked with savory mixture of lemon juice, chicken, sliced kale and chopped onions soaked in earthy bone broth. It is seasoned just with salt however black pepper can also be added as per the desired taste.

## Ingredients

- 4 cups of shredded chicken
- 6 cups bone broth
- 1 bunch of kale, rinsed, drained and sliced into 1/2 inch strips
- 3 lemons
- 2 tablespoons fresh lemon juice
- 1 cup onions, chopped
- 1/2 cup olive oil
- salt to taste

## Directions

1. Add oil, onion and 2 cups of broth to a blender and blend for 2 minutes to a get a smooth mixture.
2. Pour this mixture into the slow cooker and add all the remaining ingredients.
3. Cover the lid and cook for 6 hours on low setting.
4. Give few occasional stirs during the cooking.
5. Once done, serve warm.

## Nutrition

Calories: 393          Fats: 19.8g          Sodium: 243mg
Carbs: 5.8g          Proteins: 48g          Sugar: 1.7g

# Mexican Chicken Low Carb Soup

## Serves: 6

## Prep Time: 15mins

Enjoy the tangy flavor of chunky salsa with this scrumptious low carb Mexican soup. With the mild taste of chicken broth, spicy salsa and Pepper Jack cheese, the soup turns into a full deal for the dinner table. To reduce the hotness, the amount of salsa can be reduced as per the desired flavor.

## Ingredients

- 1 1/2 pounds chicken pieces boneless/skinless
- 15.5 ounces chunky salsa
- 15 ounces chicken broth
- 8 ounces Monterey or Pepper Jack cheese cubed small or shredded

## Directions

1. Add all thc ingrcdicnts to a 6 quart slow cooker,
2. Cover the lid and cook for 6 to 8 hours on Low or 3 to 4 hours on High setting.
3. Once done, remove the chicken from the cooker and shred it using two forks.
4. Return the shreds to the cooker and mix well.
5. Serve warm.

## Nutrition

Calories: 531        Fats: 16.2g        Sodium: 1958g

Carbs: 4.9g        Proteins: 93.9g        Sugar: 2.5g

# Low-Carb Taco Soup

**Serves: 8**

**Prep Time: 10mins**

Infuse a simple meat soup with juicy Rotel tomatoes and taco seasoning. This soup gets super rich when mixed with cream cheese and topped with shredded cheese. For a refreshing flavor add fresh cilantro to the soup and enjoy with warm bread.

## Ingredients

- 2 lbs. ground pork beef or sausage
- 2, 8- ounce packages of cream cheese
- 2, 10- ounce cans of rotel tomatoes
- 2 tablespoons of taco seasonings
- 4 cups of chicken broth
- 1-2 tablespoons of cilantro - fresh or dried optional
- 1/2 cup shredded cheese for garnish optional

## Directions

1. Sear the ground meat in a skillet over medium until brown.
2. Meanwhile, add tomatoes, taco seasoning and cream cheese to the slow cooker.
3. Transfer the meat to the cooker, leaving al the excess grease behind.
4. Add chicken broth and mix well to combine all the ingredients.
5. Cook for 4 hours on low or for 2 hours in High.
6. When the timer goes off, top the soup with shredded cheese and cilantro.
7. Serve and enjoy.

## Nutrition

Calories: 640          Fats: 54.9g          Sodium: 1653mg
Carbs: 4.1g           Proteins: 30.5g       Sugar: 1g

# Vegetable Beef Soup

**Serves: 10**

**Prep Time: 10mins**

Experience a low carb warming beef soup which is filled with range of vegetables, tomatoes, thyme and rosemary. It is loaded with bacon, beef broth, green beans, carrots, red wine and celeriac. For delayed serving, it can be refrigerated in a sealed container. Reheat on low heat for 10 minutes before serving.

## Ingredients

- 4 slices bacon sliced into 1/2 inch pieces
- 2 pounds stew meat cut into 1" cubes, patted dry
- 2 tablespoons red wine vinegar
- 32 ounces beef broth low-sodium
- 1 medium yellow onion chopped
- 1/4 cup green beans cut into 1 inch pieces
- 1 small celeriac (about 6 ounces) diced
- 1/4 cup carrots diced
- 2 tablespoons tomato paste
- 1 28 ounce can diced tomatoes
- 2 cloves garlic crushed
- 1/2 teaspoon dried rosemary
- 1/2 teaspoon dried thyme
- 1/2 teaspoon black pepper freshly ground
- 1 teaspoon sea salt

## Directions

1. Cook bacon in a skillet over medium high heat until brown and crispy.
2. Transfer the bacon to a plate, cover and refrigerate for later use.

3. Keep about 1 tablespoon of bacon grease in the pan and discard the rest.
4. Add beef cubes to the pan and cook them in batches until brown. Season the cubes with salt and pepper meanwhile.
5. Transfer the beef to the slow cooker using a slotted spoon.
6. Add vinegar to the same skillet and reduce its heat to medium low. Scrap off the brown bits.
7. Stir in 1/4 cup of broth and continue cooking with stirring for 2 minutes.
8. Transfer this mixture to the cooker and add all the remaining ingredients except for bacon.
9. Cover the lid and cook on low for 6 to 8 hours.
10. Once done, garnish with bacon and serve warm.

### Nutrition

Calories: 286

Fats: 12.9g

Sodium: 470mg

Carbs: 5.9g

Proteins: 30g

Sugar: 2.9g

# Vegetarian

## Spinach with Tomato Sauce

**Servings: 4**

**Prep Time: 7 minutes**

Spinach with tomato sauce is a creamy mixture of sautéed vegetables, cooked with the savory gravy of tomatoes, white wine and tomato puree. The crushed pepper flakes are added for a mild tangy taste.

### Ingredients
- 2 tablespoons olive oil
- 1 medium onion, chopped
- 1 tablespoon garlic, minced
- ½ teaspoon red pepper flakes, crushed
- 8 cups fresh spinach, chopped
- 1 cup tomatoes, chopped
- ½ cup homemade tomato puree
- ½ cup white wine
- ¾ cup low-sodium vegetable broth
- ½ cup cream cheese

### Directions
1. Heat oil in a skillet and sauté onions for about 3 minutes.
2. Add garlic and red pepper flakes and sauté more for 1 minute.
3. Stir in spinach and cook for 2 minutes.
4. Transfer this mixture to a greased slow cooker and add all the remaining ingredients except cheese cream.
5. Cover the lid and cook for about 3 to 4 hours on low setting.
6. Once done, mix well and top it with cream cheese.
7. Serve warm and enjoy.

### Nutrients
| | | |
|---|---|---|
| Calories: 233 | Fats: 17.5g | Sodium: 157mg |
| Carbs: 10.6g | Proteins: 5.4g | Sugar: 3.9g |

# Exotic Carrots with Mushroom Sauce

**Servings: 3**

**Prep Time: 15 minutes**

Let's endeavor the world of healthy diet and try a low carb mushroom sauce recipe which is cooked with sliced carrots. The seasoning is basic and perfectly complements the mixture of heavy cream and vegetables.

## Ingredients

- 2 tablespoons of butter
- 2 garlic cloves, minced
- 1 tablespoon of fresh sage leaves, chopped
- 1 pound fresh mushrooms, sliced
- Salt and freshly ground black pepper, to taste
- ¼ cup of heavy cream
- 1 scallion, chopped
- 3 large carrots, spiralizer with blade C
- 1 cup whipping cream

## Directions

1. Sauté garlic with basil in a skillet for 1 minute then transfer this mixture to a slow cooker.
2. Add all the remaining ingredients to the cooker.
3. Cover the lid and cook on low for 4 hours.
4. Once done, mix well and serve warm with noodles.

## Nutrition

Calories: 288

Carbs: 15g

Fats: 24.3g

Proteins: 6.8g

Sodium: 131mg

Sugar: 6.3g

# Tomato Soup

**Servings: 4**

**Prep Time: 10 minutes**

Tomato soup is one healthy and nutritious meal for your dinner table. Make you and your family a treat filled with fresh red tomatoes. Add basil and parsley for a deep earthy taste. Season with salt and pepper as per your desired taste.

## Ingredients

- ½ tablespoon olive oil
- 1 small onion, chopped
- 1 garlic clove, minced
- 1 ½ pound fresh tomatoes, chopped
- 1 tablespoon homemade tomato sauce
- 1 teaspoon dried parsley, crushed
- 1 teaspoon dried basil, crushed
- Freshly ground black pepper, to taste
- 2 cups low-sodium vegetable broth
- 2 tablespoons Erythritol
- ½ tablespoon balsamic vinegar
- ¼ cup fresh basil, chopped

## Directions

1. Heat oil in a skillet and sauté onion and garlic for about 3 minutes.
2. Transfer this mixture to a greased slow cooker.
3. Add all the remaining ingredients to the cooker except sugar, basil and vinegar.
4. Cover the lid and cook for about 1 to 2 hours on high setting.
5. Once done, mix well and stir in sugar and vinegar.
6. Use a handheld blender to puree the mixture into soup.

7. Garnish with basil and serve.

## Nutrients

| | | |
|---|---|---|
| Calories: 188 | Fats: 11.4g | Sodium: 338mg |
| Carbs: 10.2g | Proteins: 13.1g | Sugar: 5.4g |

# Cauliflower Mash

**Servings: 6**

**Prep Time: 5 minutes**

Cauliflower mash is a good and healthy alternative of popular potato mash. Allow them to steam in the slow cooker over high heat then mash the pieces together with other ingredients. Along with cheese, you can also add a bit of cream to create more variation.

## Ingredients

- 1 large head cauliflower, chop into large pieces
- 1 tablespoon butter, softened
- 1 garlic clove, minced
- ½ cup feta cheese
- 2 teaspoons fresh chives, minced
- Salt and freshly ground black pepper, to taste

## Directions

1. Fill a slow cooker with water and place the cauliflowcr picccs into it.
2. Cover the lid and let it cook for 2 to 3 hours on high setting.
3. Once done, transfer the cauliflower to a large bowl using a slotted spoon.
4. Add all the remaining ingredients to the bowl and mix well.
5. Use a potato masher or a handheld blender to blend well until the desired texture is attained.
6. Serve and enjoy.

## Nutrition

Calories: 124          Fats: 9.3g          Sodium: 333mg

Carbs: 6.1g          Proteins: 5.4g          Sugar: 3.2g

# Carrot Mash

**Servings: 4**

**Prep Time: 10 minutes**

Let's bring diversity into your menu with the delicious carrot mash. Unlike other mashed vegetables it's mildly sweet in taste and incorporates salt in a small amount. Besides these basic ingredients other varieties of spices can also be added to add variation in flavor.

## Ingredients

- 1½ pounds carrots, peeled and chopped roughly
- ½ cup butter, softened
- 1 teaspoon erythritol
- Salt, to taste

## Directions

1. Fill a slow cooker with 1 cup water and place the carrots in it.
2. Cover the lid and cook for 5 to 6 hours on high setting.
3. Once done, mash the cooked carrots with all the remaining ingredients using a hand blender.
4. Serve warm.

## Nutrition

Calories: 273

Carbs: 15g

Fats: 23g

Proteins: 1.6g

Sodium: 120mg

Sugar: 1.6g

# Rich Cheesy Broccoli Soup

**Servings: 6**

**Prep Time: 15 minutes**

There is no better way to eat broccoli than to have it in a soup full of cheese, spices and juicy vegetables. Every spoon of this will leave a rich and fulling taste in your mouth. Due to the richness of this soup it can be served at any time of the day without any side meal. However a piece of warm bread sounds delicious with it.

## Ingredients

- 1 tablespoon olive oil
- 2 tablespoons butter
- 2 medium carrots, peeled and chopped
- 1 small yellow onion, chopped
- 2 tablespoons almond flour
- 1 garlic clove, minced
- 3 cups homemade vegetable broth
- 5 cups broccoli florets
- 1 teaspoon dill weed
- 1 teaspoon smoked paprika
- Salt and freshly ground black pepper, to taste
- 4 American cheese slices, cut into pieces
- 1 cup Colby Jack cheese, shredded
- 1 cup Pepper Jack cheese, shredded
- ½ cup Parmesan cheese, shredded

## Directions

1. Heat oil in a large skillet and sauté onion and carrot in it for about 3 minutes.
2. Add garlic and flour and stir cook for 1 minute.

3. Stir in broth and cook for 1 minute with constant stirring.
4. Transfer this mixture to the slow cooker and add broccoli into it.
5. Cover the lid and cook for about 5 to 6 hours on high setting.
6. Once done, add salt, pepper, paprika, dill, milk and cheeses to the broccoli. Mix well
7. Serve warm and enjoy.

## Nutrients

Calories: 354

Fats: 26.1g

Sodium: 874mg

Carbs: 12.9g

Proteins: 18.8g

Sugar: 4.9g

# Nutty Brussels Sprout

**Servings: 3**

**Preparation Time: 10 minutes**

This three ingredient Brussels sprout recipe is so simple and east to make. Just steam the trimmed vegetable in the slow cooker and then serve it with the nutty almond topping and melted butter. Serve fresh for best flavor.

## Ingredients

- 1 pound Brussels sprouts, trimmed and halve
- ¼ cup butter, melted
- ½ cup almonds, chopped

## Directions

1. Add water to the slow cooker, just enough to cover its base.
2. Place the Brussels sprout in it and cover the lid to cook for 6 hours on low setting.
3. Once done, transfer them onto a serving plate.
4. Top them with melted butter and almonds.
5. Serve warm and fresh.

## Nutrition

Calories: 293          Fats: 23.8g          Sodium: 147mg

Carbs: 14.2g          Proteins: 8.7g          Sugar: 3.9g

# Stunning Broccoli Florets

**Servings: 6**

**Prep Time: 15 minutes**

These broccoli florets are steamed through slow cooking without any spices. Once cooked the broccolis are served fresh with the creamy seasoned mixture and melted butter. Pair these florets with mixed vegetable rice or pasta of your choice.

## Ingredients

- 2 pounds broccoli florets
- 4 tablespoons butter, melted
- 1 cup whipping cream
- Salt and freshly ground black pepper, to taste

## Directions

1. Add water to the slow cooker, just enough to cover its base.
2. Place the broccoli floret in it and cover the lid to cook for 6 hours on low setting.
3. Once done, transfer them onto a serving plate.
4. Top them with melted butter, cream, salt and pepper.
5. Serve warm and fresh.

## Nutrition

Calories: 178      Fats: 14.4g      Sodium: 111mg

Carbs: 10.6g      Proteins: 4.7g      Sugar: 2.6g

# Veggies Dish

**Servings: 4**

**Prep Time: 10 minutes**

A full vegetable package is set to make your dinner table even more tempting. Zucchini, a vegetable of great taste and nutrition is added to this stew which is slow cooked with mushrooms and tomatoes. Top the dish with the mixture of cheeses and allow them to melt before serving.

## Ingredients

- 6-ounce fresh mushrooms, sliced
- ½ cup onion, chopped
- 2 zucchinis, cut into ½-inch slices
- 1 tablespoons fresh basil, chopped
- ½ tablespoon olive oil
- ½ cup cream
- ½ cup cheddar cheese
- ½ cup feta cheese
- 1 garlic cloves, minced
- Salt and freshly ground black pepper, to taste
- ½ (7-ounce) can sugar-free crushed tomatoes with juice

## Directions

1. Heat oil in a large skillet and sauté onion, garlic and mushrooms for about 5 minutes.
2. Add basil and zucchini and sauté more for 1 minute.
3. Transfer this mixture to a greased slow cooker.
4. Add all the remaining ingredients to the cooker except all the cheeses and mix well.
5. Cover the lid and cook for about 4 to 5 hours on high setting.

6. Once done, mix well and top it with all the cheeses. Let it stay to melt.

7. Serve warm and enjoy.

## Nutrition

Calories: 306          Fats: 14.3g          Sodium: 482mg

Carbs: 7.9g          Proteins: 18.7g          Sugar: 4g

# Cheesy Cauliflower

**Servings: 5**

**Prep Time: 5 minutes**

Cauliflower has its own distinctive taste and aroma, so when it is cooked with these basic ingredients in a slow cooker, the vegetables blends with an appealing taste. Cheese and butter used in the recipe, is great for people of young ages.

## Ingredients

- 1 head cauliflower
- 1 tablespoon prepared mustard
- 1 teaspoon mayonnaise
- ¼ cup butter, cut into small pieces
- ½ cup Parmesan cheese, grated

## Directions

1. Grease your slow cooker with butter.

2. Add all the ingredients to the cooker and mix them well.

3. Cover the lid and cook on high got 2 to 3 hours.

4. Once done, give a few stirs then serve.

## Nutrition

Calories: 155

Carbs: 3.8g

Fats: 13.3g

Proteins: 6.7g

Sodium: 280mg

Sugar: 1.4g

# Side Dishes

## Warm Chicken Nacho Dip

**Servings: 12**

**Prep Time: 20 minutes**

A tasty dip is essential to pair with a complete meal and or with a delicious evening snack. And this healthy and nutritious chicken dip will serve that purpose. Serve with fresh vegetable salad or any other snack of your choice, it will taste equally filling.

### Ingredients

- 1 (14 ounce) can diced tomatoes with green Chile peppers, drained
- 1 (1 pound) loaf processed cheese food, cubed
- 2 large cooked skinless, boneless chicken breast halves, shredded
- 1/3 cup sour cream
- 1/4 cup diced green onion
- 1 1/2 tablespoons taco seasoning mix
- 2 tablespoons minced jalapeno pepper, or to taste

### Directions

1. Add all the ingredients to the slow cooker.
2. Cover the lid and cook for about 1 to 2 hours on high with occasional stirring.
3. Once done, mix well and serve as a dip

### Nutrients

Calories: 232     Fats: 13.6g     Sodium: 790mg

Carbs: 8.7g     Proteins: 18.6g     Sugar: 1.6g

# Little Smokies

**Servings: 16**

**Prep Time: 10 minutes**

Barbeque sauce glazed sausages are perfect to complement a light dinner or a supper. The sausages are dipped and cooked in the blend of tangy and sweet sauces along with chopped onions. For best serving, serve the Smokies with a wooden stick stuck in the center.

## Ingredients

- 1 (18 ounce) bottle barbeque sauce
- 1 cup honey
- 1/2 cup sugar free tomato sauce
- 1 tablespoon Worcestershire sauce
- 1/3 cup chopped onion
- 2 (16 ounce) packages little wieners

## Directions

1. add all the ingredients to the cooker and mix well.

2. Cover and cook on low for 2 hours.

3. Serve and enjoy.

## Nutrition

Calories: 285          Fats: 16.4g          Sodium: 599mg

Carbs: 28.6g          Proteins: 19.7g          Sugar: 1.1g

# Marinated Mushrooms

**Servings: 12**

**Prep Time: 3 minutes**

We all know how delicious and healthy mushrooms are, perhaps it is the most popular ingredient of western cuisine. With this marinated mushroom recipe, now we can enjoy fresh mushrooms with juicy mix of bouillon with wine and Worcestershire sauce.

## Ingredients

- 4 cubes chicken bouillon
- 4 cubes beef bouillon
- 2 cups boiling water
- 1 cup dry red wine
- 1 teaspoon dill weed
- 1 teaspoon Worcestershire sauce
- 1 teaspoon garlic powder
- 4 pounds fresh mushrooms
- 1/2 cup butter, or more as needed

## Directions

1. Add bouillon cubes to the boiling water and mix well. Stir in red wine, dill, garlic powder and Worcestershire sauce.
2. Place the mushrooms in the slow cooker and top them with prepared mixture.
3. Add butter on top and cook on low for 12 hours.
4. Mix and serve warm.

## Nutrients

Calories: 124          Fats: 8.3g          Sodium: 741mg

Carbs: 6.4g          Proteins: 5.3g          Sugar: 1.2g

# Cowboy Mexican Dip

**Servings: 24**

**Prep Time: 10 minutes**

It's about time, to prepare a tangy Mexican dip which is loaded with processed cheese and tomatoes. With simple ingredients and special beef tamales, this delectable dip gets more filling and nourishing. The melts slowly during the cooking and blends well with all the ingredients of the dip.

## Ingredients

- 12 beef tamales, husked and mashed
- 1 (15 ounce) can chili without beans
- 1 (14.5 ounce) can diced tomatoes and green chiles
- 1 (1 pound) loaf processed cheese, cubed

## Directions

1. Add cheese, tamales, tomatoes and chili to the slow cooker.
2. Cook on high setting until the cheese melts.
3. Once done, mix well and serve.

## Nutrition

Calories: 117          Fats: 7.5g          Sodium: 447mg

Carbs: 7.2g          Proteins: 5.7g          Sugar: 1.4g

# Glazed Spiced Carrots

**Servings: 6**

**Prep Time: 10 minutes**

Carrots, the known source of vitamin A, fibers and minerals, are the best vegetables to side your main course with. Unlike fresh salads, these glazed carrots are coated with the mixture of sugar and spices then topped with crunchy pecans.

## Ingredients
- 2 pounds small carrots
- 1/2 cup peach preserves
- 1/2 cup butter, melted
- 1/4 cup packed brown sugar
- 1 teaspoon vanilla extract
- 1/2 teaspoon ground cinnamon
- 1/4 teaspoon salt
- 1/8 teaspoon ground nutmeg
- 2 tablespoons cornstarch
- 2 tablespoons water
- Toasted chopped pecans, optional

## Directions
1. Mix butter with salt, nutmeg, vanilla, butter and brown sugar in a bowl and keep it aside.
2. Dissolve cornstarch in water and pour it into the nutmeg mixture. Mix well to combine.
3. Place the carrots in a 3 quart slow cooker and pour the prepared sauce on top.
4. Cover the lid and cook on low for about 6 to 8 hours.
5. Once done, top the carrots with pecans and serve.

## Nutrition
Calories: 391

Carbs: 9.2g

Fats: 23g

Proteins: 34.9g

Sodium: 577mg

Sugar: 7.5g

# Italian Mushrooms

**Servings: 6**

**Prep Time: 10 minutes**

The Italian mushrooms are seasoned generously with Italian salad dressing and rich melted butter. This simple 4 ingredients recipe is completely effortless, just add ingredients together than slow cook them for hours until the vegetable are al dente.

## Ingredients

- 1 pound medium fresh mushrooms
- 1 large onion, sliced
- 1/2 cup butter, melted
- 1 envelope Italian salad dressing mix

## Directions

1. Add onion and mushrooms to a 3 quart slow cooker.
2. Mix butter with salad dressing mix in a small bowl.
3. Pour this mixture over the vegetables and mix well.
4. Cover the lid and cook for 4 to 5 hours on low.
5. Serve warm and enjoy.

## Nutrients

Calories: 417          Fats: 27.7g          Sodium: 626mg

Carbs: 12.2g          Proteins: 18.5g          Sugar: 1.6g

# Garlic Green Beans with Gorgonzola

**Servings: 10**

**Preparation Time: 20 minutes**

Have fresh green beans cooked with mixture of sour cream, cheese, chestnuts and simple spices. Once cooked the scrumptious beans are topped with crispy bacon to add some extra crunch. Keep it warm then serve and enjoy with your favorite meal.

## Ingredients

- 2 pounds fresh green beans, trimmed and halved
- 1 can (8 ounces) sliced water chestnuts, drained
- 4 green onions, chopped
- 5 bacon strips, cooked and crumbled, divided
- 1/3 cup white wine or chicken broth
- 2 tablespoons minced fresh thyme or 2 teaspoons dried thyme
- 4 garlic cloves, minced
- 1-1/2 teaspoons seasoned salt
- 1 cup (8 ounces) sour cream
- 3/4 cup crumbled Gorgonzola cheese

## Directions

1. Add water, green beans, green onions, chestnuts and 1/4 cup bacon to a 4 quart slow cooker.
2. Mix wine with garlic, salt and thyme in a small bowl.
3. Pour this mixture over the vegetables in the cooker.
4. Cover the lid and cook for about 3 to 4 hours on low.
5. Drain the excessive liquid and serve warm with cheese and bacon on top.

## Nutrition

Calories: 225          Fats: 11.2g          Sodium: 471mg
Carbs: 6.5g           Proteins: 25.5g      Sugar: 3.1g

# Slow-Cooked Green Beans

**Servings: 12**

**Prep Time: 10 minutes**

Another low carb, slow cooker recipe for green beans is here. These special French style green beans are cooked with melted butter, soy sauce, garlic salt and earthy brown sugar. Let them cook together on low for some hours the mix and serve.

## Ingredients

- 16 cups frozen French-style green beans (about 48 ounces), thawed
- 1/2 cup butter, melted
- 1/2 cup packed brown sugar
- 1-1/2 teaspoons garlic salt
- 3/4 teaspoon reduced-sodium soy sauce

## Directions

1. Spread the green beans in the slow cooker.
2. Mix all the remaining ingredients in a bowl and pour that mixture over the beans.
3. Cover the lid and cook for 2 to 3 hours on low.
4. Once done, mix well and enjoy.

## Nutrition

| | | |
|---|---|---|
| Calories: 160 | Fats: 7.1g | Sodium: 428mg |
| Carbs: 11.3g | Proteins: 11.2g | Sugar: 1.1g |

# Party Sausages

**Servings: 16**

**Prep Time: 5 minutes**

a distinct flavor of these party sausages will inspire you with its juicy pineapple taste along with the aroma of its Catalina and Russian dressing. Together these ingredients creates an inspiring blend. To serve always garnish with fresh chopped green onions.

## Ingredients

- 2 pounds smoked sausage links, sliced diagonally
- 1 bottle (8 ounces) Catalina salad dressing
- 1 bottle (8 ounces) Russian salad dressing
- 1/2 cup packed brown sugar
- 1/2 cup pineapple juice
- Sliced green onions, optional

## Direction

1. Sear the sausages in a skillet until brown then transfer them to a 3 quart slow cooker.
2. Mix all the remaining ingredients a small bowl and pour this mixture over the sausages.
3. Cover the lid and cook for 1 to 2 hours on low.
4. Garnish with green onions and serve warm.

## Nutrition

Calories: 326        Fats: 25g        Sodium: 924mg

Carbs: 15g        Proteins: 7g        Sugar: 17g

# Collard Greens

**Servings: 16**

**Prep Time: 30 minutes**

The cauliflower combine with cheese gives a perfect dish on your table.

## Ingredients

- 4 bunches collard greens - rinsed, trimmed and chopped
- 1 pound ham shanks
- 4 pickled jalapeno peppers, chopped
- 1/2 teaspoon baking soda
- 1 teaspoon olive oil
- ground black pepper to taste
- garlic powder to taste

## Directions

1. Fill a large saucepan with water upto ½ full then add ham and greens in it.
2. Bring the water to a boil. Then immediately transfer the greens to a bowl using a slotted spoon.
3. Add a layer of greens then ham shanks and jalapeno into the slow cooker.
4. Mix olive oil, pepper and garlic powder in a small bowl.
5. Pour this mixture into the slow cooker.
6. Cover and cook on low for 8 to 10 hours.
7. Once done, mix well and serve.

## Nutrition

| | | |
|---|---|---|
| Calories: 99 | Fats: 6.6g | Sodium: 82mg |
| Carbs: 4.2g | Proteins: 6.6g | Sugar: 0.1g |

# Seafood

## Flavorsome Fish Curry

**Servings: 3**

**Prep Time: 15 minutes**

A low budget, low carb and extremely delicious fish curry is what we all long for. The addition of variety of new spices to the basic fish recipe adds a unique blended flavor. The salmon fillets are soaked and slow cooked in the aromatic curry mixture.

### Ingredients

- 1 pound salmon fillets, cut into bite sized pieces
- 1 curry leaves
- ½ tablespoon olive oil
- ½ teaspoon red chili powder½ small yellow onion, chopped
- 1 garlic cloves, minced
- 1 tablespoons curry powder
- 1 teaspoons ground cumin
- 1 teaspoons ground coriander
- ½ teaspoon ground turmeric
- 1 cup unsweetened coconut milk
- 1 cups tomatoes, chopped
- ½ Serrano pepper, seeded and chopped
- ½ tablespoon fresh lemon juice

### Directions

1. Preheat the slow cooker on high settings.

2. Add curry leaves, garlic and onions to stir cook for 4 to 5 minutes.

3. Stir in all the remaining ingredients to the cooker.

4. Cover the lid and cook for 1 to 2 hours on High setting.

5. Once done, drizzle some lemon juice on top.
6. Serve warm and enjoy.

**Nutrients**

| | | |
|---|---|---|
| Calories: 441 | Fats: 31.7g | Sodium: 91mg |
| Carbs: 11.5g | Proteins: 32.7g | Sugar: 5g |

# Elegant Dinner Mussels

## Servings: 6
## Prep Time: 20 minutes

Mussels, when cooked with lemony mixture of spices, tastes amazingly. Before adding the mussles to the cooker, make sure they are properly cleaned and scrapped from outside then place them gently into the cooker.

## Ingredients
- 2 pounds mussels, cleaned and de-bearded
- 2 tablespoons butter
- 1 medium yellow onion, chopped
- 1 garlic clove, minced
- ½ teaspoon dried rosemary, crushed
- 1 cup homemade chicken broth
- 2 tablespoons fresh lemon juice
- ½ cup sour cream
- Salt and freshly ground black pepper, to taste

## Directions:
1. Add all ingredients to the slow cooker except sour cream.
2. Cover the lid and cook on high for 1 hour.
3. When the timer goes off, mix well and transfer the mixture to a serving bowl.
4. Top with sour cream and serve.

## Nutrition
Calories: 221     Fats: 11.6g     Sodium: 599mg

Carbs: 8.6g     Proteins: 19.7g     Sugar: 1.1g

# Lobster Dinner

**Servings: 2**

**Prep Time: 3 minutes**

Lobster meat does not only tastes good, but it is also rich in good proteins and fats. Lobster tails are one the of most famous seafood which is served at almost every other home and the restaurant. Well, now you can too, prepare it so easily using your own slow cooker.

## Ingredients

- 2 pounds lobster tails, cut in half
- 2 tablespoons unsalted butter, melted
- Pinch of salt
- 2 oz. white wine
- 4 oz. Water

## Directions

1. Add all the liquids to the slow cooker.

2. Place the lobstcr tail in it.

3. Cover the lid and cook on low for 10 minutes.

4. Once done, let it stay for 5 minutes then serve.

5. Season with salt and butter then serve.

## Nutrients

Calories: 169          Fats: 5.1g          Sodium: 762mg

Carbs: 0g          Proteins: 28.8g          Sugar: 0g

# Curried Shrimp

**Servings: 5**

**Prep Time: 10 minutes**

Curried shrimps are great for a weekend luncheon. Prepare a hot and comforting bowl of shrimp curry and serve it with steaming brown rice or with some side salad. The seasoning can also be adjusted as per the desired taste.

## Ingredients

- 1 tablespoon olive oil
- 1 medium onion, chopped
- ½ teaspoon ground cumin
- 1½ teaspoons red chili powder
- 1 teaspoon ground turmeric
- Pinch of salt
- 2 medium tomatoes, chopped
- ¼ cup water
- 1¾ pounds medium shrimp, peeled and deveined
- 1 tablespoon fresh lemon juice
- ¼ cup fresh cilantro, chopped

## Directions

1. Add all the ingredients to the slow cooker except the shrimps.
2. Cover and cook on low for 2 hours.
3. Once done, remove the lid and stir in shrimps.
4. Cook for 30 minutes on low.
5. Once done, mix well and serve.

## Nutrition

Calories: 328

Carbs: 4.9g

Fats: 6.7g

Proteins: 64.1g

Sodium: 711mg

Sugar: 2.4g

# Lemon Salmon

**Servings: 3**

**Prep Time: 7 minutes**

Have a bite of a juicy salmon fillets, which are simply seasoned with salt and pepper. However the flavor gets more inviting when the fillets are cooked with lemon slices, aromatic vegetables or herbs. Once steamed the fillets can be served with creamy salads or dips.

## Ingredients

- 1 to 2 pounds skin-on salmon fillets
- Salt, to taste
- Fresh ground black pepper
- Sliced lemon (optional)
- Sliced aromatic vegetables, like fennel, onions, or celery (optional)
- 1 to 1 1/2 cups liquid, such as water, broth, wine, beer, cider, or a mix

## Directions

1. Line the inside of your slow cooker with aluminum foil.
2. Place the salmon fillets in it. Top them with herbs, lemon, liquid and seasoning.
3. Cover the lid of cooker and cook for about 1 to 2 hours on Low.
4. Once done, remove the fish from the cooker.
5. Garnish with lemon slices and serve.

## Nutrition

Calories: 391          Fats: 23g          Sodium: 577mg

Carbs: 9.2g          Proteins: 34.9g          Sugar: 7.5g

# Seafood Stew

**Servings: 4**

**Prep Time: 10 minutes**

Prepare a seafood delight with fresh shrimps and scallops with this simple stew recipe. First slow cook the curry using crushed tomatoes and tomato paste then add seafood to the mixture. The slower you cook, the better flavor they get.

## Ingredients

- 1 can (28 oz.) crushed tomatoes
- 1 Tablespoon tomato paste
- 4 cups vegetable broth
- 3 garlic cloves, minced
- 1/2 cup chopped white onion
- 1 teaspoon dried thyme
- 1 teaspoon dried basil
- 1 teaspoon dried oregano
- 1/2 teaspoon celery salt
- 1/4 teaspoon crush red pepper flakes
- 1/8 teaspoon cayenne pepper
- salt and pepper to taste
- 2 pounds seafood (1 pound large shrimp and 1 pound scallops)
- handful of chopped parsley

## Directions

1. Add all the ingredients to the slow cooker except seafood and parsley.
2. Cover the lid and cook for 2 to 3 hours on high.
3. Once done, remove the lid and add the seafood to the mixture.
4. Cook for another 30 to 60 minutes until seafood is al dente.

5. Garnish with parsley and serve.

## Nutrients

| | | |
|---|---|---|
| Calories: 417 | Fats: 27.7g | Sodium: 626mg |
| Carbs: 12.2g | Proteins: 18.5g | Sugar: 1.6g |

# Omega-3 Rich Salmon Soup

**Servings: 4**

**Preparation Time: 15 minutes**

Omega 3 is essential for our body and provides basic nutrients for growth and nourishment. And this soup is a perfect source of omega 3, as it is made out of salmon. The salmon is paired with a mix of juicy vegetables and is slow cooked in the broth.

## Ingredients

- 1 pound salmon fillets
- 1 tablespoon coconut oil
- 1 cups carrots, peeled and chopped
- ½ cup celery stalk, chopped
- ½ cup yellow onion, chopped
- 1 cup cauliflower, chopped
- 2 cups homemade chicken broth
- Salt and freshly ground black pepper, to taste
- ¼ cup fresh parsley, chopped

## Directions

1. Line the slow cooker with aluminum foil and add 1 cup water into it.
2. Place the salmon fillets in it and cover the lid to cook for 1 to 2 hours on low.
3. When the timer goes, transfer the fish to a plate and empty the cooker.
4. Add all the remaining ingredients to the cooker and cook for about 3 to 4 hours on high.
5. Return the fish to the cooker and flip to coat it well.
6. Serve warm.

## Nutrition

Calories: 225

Fats: 11.2g

Sodium: 471mg

Carbs: 6.5g

Proteins: 25.5g

Sugar: 3.1g

# Citrus Glazed Salmon

**Servings: 2**

**Prep Time: 10 minutes**

When salmon is cooked in a juicy mix of whine and orange juice, you get a delicious citrus glazed salmon for your tables. Add salt and pepper for some seasoning and cook with ginger for a defining and tempting aroma.

## Ingredients

- 2 (4-ounce) salmon fillets
- ½ teaspoon fresh ginger, minced
- 1 teaspoon fresh orange zest, grated finely
- ½ cup white wine
- ½ tablespoon olive oil
- 1 tablespoon fresh orange juice
- freshly ground black pepper, to taste

## Directions

1. Add all the ingredients to the slow cooker and mix gently.

2. Cover the lid and cook for 1 hour on low setting.

3. When the timer goes off, transfer the fillets to the serving plate.

4. Top the fish with it sauce and serve warm.

## Nutrition

| | | |
|---|---|---|
| Calories: 160 | Fats: 7.1g | Sodium: 28mg |
| Carbs: 3g | Proteins: 11.2g | Sugar: 1.1g |

# Cod & Peas with Sour Cream

**Servings: 2**

**Prep Time: 5 minutes**

Here is a fine combination of seafood and veggies. The cod fillets are cooked with parsley and peas with the blend of garlic and paprika. As the white wine is added during the cooking, it absorbs into the fish, rendering it even more tasty.

## Ingredients

- 2 (4-ounce) cod fillets
- 1 tablespoon fresh parsley
- 1 garlic clove, chopped
- ½ pound frozen peas
- ½ teaspoon paprika
- 1 cup sour cream
- ½ cup white wine

## Direction

1. Line the slow cooker with aluminum foil and add place the cod fillets in it.
2. Add all the remaining ingredients except the sour cream.
3. Cover the lid and cook for about 2 hours on high setting.
4. Once done, transfer the fillets to the plate.
5. Top it with remaining pea's mixture and sour cream.
6. Serve and enjoy.

## Nutrition

Calories: 385

Carbs: 11g

Fats: 25g

Proteins: 19.8g

Sodium: 180mg

Sugar: 5.5g

# Nutritious Salmon Dinner

**Servings: 2**

**Prep Time: 10 minutes**

Let's prepare simple salmon for the meal with the inspiring new recipe. The fish is first seasoned and then cooked in the liquid. For better flavor, the fish can also be marinated in the refrigerator using a sealed container. The longer the marination the better the taste will be.

## Ingredients

- 1 pound salmon fillet, cut into 3 pieces
- 1 garlic clove, minced
- 1 teaspoon powdered stevia
- 1 tablespoon red chili powder
- 1 teaspoon ground cumin
- Salt and freshly ground black pepper
- ½ cup red wine
- ½ cup broth

## Directions

1. Mix all the spices in a bowl and season the fish with this rub.
2. Line the slow cooker with aluminum foil and add the wine and broth in it.
3. Place the seasoned fish in it.
4. Cover the lid and cook for 2 to 3 hours on low.
5. Once done, transfer the fish to a plate and garnish with fresh herbs.
6. Serve warm and enjoy.

## Nutrition

Calories: 212

Fats: 9.7g

Sodium: 93mg

Carbs: 2g

Proteins: 29.8g

Sugar: 0.2g

# Beverages

## Viennese Coffee Recipe

**Serves: 4**

**Prep Time: 5 mins**

Prepare a soothing Viennese coffee with a twist of keto style. It is pure mixture of brewed coffee, chocolate syrup and stevia which are cooked together for a nice blend. Once prepared, the coffee is served with rich cream toppings.

### Ingredients

- 3 cups strong brewed coffee
- 3 tablespoons sugar free chocolate syrup
- 1 teaspoon stevia
- 1/3 cup heavy whipping cream
- 1/4 cup crème de cacao or Irish cream liqueur
- Whipped cream, optional

### Directions

1. Mix coffee with stevia and chocolate syrup in a 1.5 quart slow cooker.
2. Cover the lid and cook for about 2.5 hours on Low.
3. Once done, pour the coffee into the serving cups and top it with Irish cream and whipped cream.
4. Serve warm or chilled, as desired.

### Nutrition

Calories: 144         Fats: 7.1g          Sodium: 31mg

Carbs: 9.6g          Proteins: 0.7g      Sugar: 8.2g

# Ginger Tea Drink Recipe

**Serves: 6**

**Prep Time: 5 mins**

Green tea is great to activate your metabolism and helps the body loose excess fats and toxin, moreover gingerroot is a known cure to all the digestive or other disorder.    When cooked together in a tea, their blend makes a refreshing new beverage which will detoxify your body and leave you fresh and lovely.

## Ingredients

- 4 cups boiling water
- 15 individual green tea bags
- 4 cups white grape juice
- 1 to 2 tablespoons honey
- 1 tablespoon minced fresh gingerroot
- Crystallized ginger, optional

## Directions

1.   Fill a 3 quart slow cooker with boiling water and place tea bags in it.
2. Cover the lid and let it stay for 10 minutes then discard the tea bags.
3. Add all the remaining ingredients to the cooker and cover the lid to cook on low for 2 to 3 hours.
4. When the timer goes off, strain this mixture and pour into the serving glasses.
5. Garnish with ginger and serve warm or chilled (as desired)

## Nutrition

Calories: 51                    Carbs: 12g                    Fats: 0.2g

Proteins: 0.7g          Sodium: 5mg          Sugar: 11.3g

# Hot Spiced Wine Recipe

**Serves: 6**

**Prep Time: 5 mins**

Get cup of hot spice wine with hints of cinnamon and apple juice on a special weeknight. Red wine is slow cooked for hours with apple and sugar free juices for juices to get this beverage done. Addition of lemon juice gives this drink a sour and savory touch.

## Ingredients

- 2 cinnamon sticks (3 inches)
- 3 whole cloves
- 3 medium tart apples, peeled and sliced
- 1/2 cup stevia
- 2 cups sugar free apple juice
- 1 teaspoon lemon juice
- 2 bottles (750 milliliters each) dry red wine

## Directions

1. Tie the cinnamon sticks and cloves in a double layered cheesecloth.
2. Place this spice bag in a 3 quart slow cooker and add all the remaining ingredients.
3. Cover the lid and cook for 4 to 5 hours on Low.
4. Once done, discard the spice bag and pour the spiced wine into the cups.
5. Serve warm or chilled.

## Nutrients

Calories: 66

Carbs: 7.9g

Fats: 0.2g

Proteins: 0.3g

Sodium: 3mg

Sugar: 8.9g

# Sweet Kahlua Coffee Recipe

**Serves: 6**

**Prep Time:    5mins**

Sweet Kahlua is on the Keto menu today, due to its new slow cooker recipe. The recipe is distinct in taste and the combination of creamy, rich, and sugar free ingredients. While preparing this coffee, go for the special sugar free chocolate chips else use any other favorite topping of yours.

## Ingredients
- 2 quarts hot water
- 1/2 cup Kahlua (coffee liqueur)
- 1/4 cup crème de cacao
- 3 tablespoons instant coffee granules
- 2 cups heavy whipping cream
- 1/4 cup stevia
- 1 teaspoon vanilla extract
- 2 tablespoons sugar free chocolate chips

## Directions
1. Fill a 4 quart slow cooker with water and add Kalua, coffee granules and crème de cacao to the cooker.
2. Cover the lid and cook for 3 to 4 hours on low.
3. Beat cream in a large bowl until it thickens. Add vanilla and stevia then beat again until foamy.
4. When the coffee is done, pour it into the serving cups and top it with whipped cream and chocolate chips.
5. Chill well before serving.

## Nutrition
Calories: 202          Fats: 12g          Sodium: 21mg
Carbs: 11.7g          Proteins: 0.8g          Sugar: 2.3g

# Slow Cooker Milk Tea Recipe

**Serves: 12**

**Prep Time: 10mins**

This one is traditional eastern tea, which is enjoy with the essence of black tea, mixed with warm milk. Along with these basic ingredients it is also loaded with the enticing flavor of gingerroot, cardamom and peppercorns. The drink is perfect to refresh you in the morning.

## Ingredients

- 15 slices fresh gingerroot (about 3 ounces)
- 3 cinnamon sticks (3 inches)
- 25 whole cloves
- 15 cardamom pods, lightly crushed
- 3 whole peppercorns
- 3-1/2 quarts water
- 8 black tea bags
- 1 cup evaporated milk
- 2 tablespoons stevia

## Directions

1. Tie the cloves, peppercorns, cardamom, cinnamon and gingerroot in a thick cheesecloth.
2. Place the bag in a 5 to 6 quart slow cooker then pour the water into it.
3. Cover and cook on low for 8 hours then discard the spice bag.
4. Add tea bags to the hot water and let it stay for 3 to 5 minutes while covering the lid.
5. Discard tea bags and add milk to the tea.
6. Serve warm in the serving cups.

## Nutrition

Calories: 25          Fats: 1g          Sodium: 20mg

Carbs: 3.3g          Proteins: 0.8g          Sugar: 1.1g

# Spiced Lemon Drink

**Serves: 12**

**Prep Time: 5mins**

Discover the refreshing flavor of this inspiring lemon drink which is mix with nourishing orange and pineapple juice. Due to its sweet and soothing juice the drink is a must have for blazing summer days. Essence of strong spices like cinnamon and cloves is also added to the recipe to help detox your body and mind.

## Ingredients

- 2-1/2 quarts water
- 2 cups stevia
- 1-1/2 cups orange juice
- 1/2 cup plus 2 tablespoons lemon juice
- 1/4 cup pineapple juice
- 1 cinnamon stick (3 inches)
- 1/2 teaspoon whole cloves

## Directions

1. Fill a 5 quart slow cooker with water, juices and sugar.
2. Tie the cinnamon and cloves in a thick cheesecloth and place it in the cooker.
3. Cover the lid and cook for 2 to 3 hours on Low.
4. Once done, discard the spice bad and pour the drink into the cups.
5. Serve warm or chill.

## Nutrients

Calories: 12

Fats: 0.2g

Sodium: 6mg

Carbs: 7.1g

Proteins: 0.4g

Sugar: 8g

# Truffle Hot Chocolate Recipe

**Serves: 6**

**Prep Time: 10 mins**

Truffle hot chocolate is everyone's favorite, for its milky chocolate taste, boosted by the strong flavor of expresso. A mild vanilla flavor is also there to tempt you but the most inspiring is the Irish topping which is a foamy mixture of Irish liqueur and cream.

## Ingredients

- 4 cups 2% milk
- 6 ounces 70% cacao dark baking chocolate, chopped
- 3 tablespoons stevia
- 1 teaspoon instant espresso powder
- 1 teaspoon vanilla extract
- Dash salt
- For Irish Whipped Cream:
- 1/2 cup heavy whipping cream
- 1 tablespoon Irish cream liqueur

## Directions

1. Add milk, cacao chocolate, and stevia, expresso, vanilla and salt to the slow cooker and mix well.
2. Cover the lid and cook for 2 hours on low. Stir well after every 15 minutes.
3. Meanwhile beat cream with Irish cream liqueur in a bowl.
4. Once done, transfer the hot chocolate to the serving cup and top it with Irish whipped cream.
5. Serve warm.

## Nutrition

Calories: 171        Fats: 11g        Sodium: 116mg
Carbs: 13.5g        Proteins: 6.2g        Sugar: 10.1g

# Mulled Merlot

**Serves: 9**

**Prep Time: 5mins**

Try a brandy filled juicy mix of orange and merlot. Cook them together slowly for an hour to make a refreshing drink for weekend nights. This spice drink is also great to serve at home parties or other festive occasion.

## Ingredients

- 4 cinnamon sticks (3 inches)
- 4 whole cloves
- 2 bottles (750 milliliters each) merlot
- 1/2 cup stevia
- 1/2 cup orange juice
- 1/2 cup brandy
- 1 medium orange, thinly sliced

## Direction

1. Tie the cinnamon sticks and cloves in a thick cheesecloth and place it in a 3 quart slow cooker.
2. Add all the ingredients to the cooker and cover the lid to cook for 1 hour on high setting.
3. When the timer goes off, discard the spice bag then transfer the drink to the serving cups.
4. Garnish with orange slices and serve.

## Nutrition

| | | |
|---|---|---|
| Calories: 59 | Fats: 0.2g | Sodium: 3mg |
| Carbs: 5.6g | Proteins: 0.3g | Sugar: 3.1g |

# Spiced Ambrosia Punch Recipe

**Serves: 8**

**Prep Time: 10mins**

Spiced ambrosia punch gives you a dose of refreshing lemon juice, apricot nectar and apple juice, all blended well into a single drink along with the essence of gingerroot, nutmeg, orange peel and cinnamon sticks. If desired, chill well for 30 minutes in the refrigerator then serve.

## Ingredients
- 3-1/2 cups sugar free apple juice
- 3 cups apricot nectar
- 1/4 cup water
- 3 tablespoons lemon juice
- 1/2 teaspoon ground cardamom
- 1/2 teaspoon ground nutmeg
- 2 cinnamon sticks (3 inches)
- 1 teaspoon finely chopped fresh gingerroot
- 1 teaspoon grated orange peel
- 8 whole cloves
- Orange slices and lemon peel strips, optional

## Directions
1. Tie the ginger, orange peel and cinnamon sticks in a cheesecloth and place it in a 3 to 4 quart slow cooker.
2. Add the remaining ingredients to the cooker and cover the lid to cook for 3 to 4 hours on Low.
3. Discard the spice bag and pour the drink into the serving cups.
4. Garnish with lemon peel and orange slices.

## Nutrition
Calories: 53

Carbs: 13.2g

Fats: 0.3g

Proteins: 0.5g

Sodium: 49mg

Sugar: 1.4g

# Slow-Cooked Apple Cranberry Cider

**Serves: 11**

**Prep Time: 10mins**

Cranberries are a good source vitamin C, E and k, along with many other essential minerals. So this cranberry cider is one healthy energy drink which can give a kicking start to your day. Once prepared, the cider can be stored in the refrigerated for a day or two.

## Ingredients

- 3 cinnamon sticks (3 inches), broken
- 1 teaspoon whole cloves
- 2 quarts sugar free apple juice
- 3 cups cranberry juice
- 2 tablespoons stevia

## Directions

1. Tie the cloves and cinnamon sticks in a thick cheesecloth and place it in a 5 quart slow cooker.
2. Add all the remaining ingredients to the cooker and cover the lid to cook for 2 hours on high setting.
3. Once done, discard the spice bag and serve in the cups.

## Nutrition

Calories: 19

Carbs: 3.4g

Fats: 0.1g

Proteins: 0g

Sodium: 41mg

Sugar: 1.1g

# Desserts

## Sugar-Free Dairy Free Fudge

**Serves: 30**

**Prep Time: 5 mins**

Dessert lovers, it's time to get excited for a sugar free keto treat full of milk and chocolate. Put all your worries behind and make yourself this delicious fudge which slow cooked with a blend of vanilla extract, stevia and salt.

### Ingredients

- 2 1/2 cups sugar-free chocolate chips
- 1/3 cup coconut milk
- 1 teaspoons pure vanilla extract
- a dash of salt
- 2 teaspoons vanilla liquid stevia (optional).

### Directions

1. Add all the ingredients to a 3 to 4 quart slow cooker and mix them together.
2. Cover the lid and cook on low for about 2 hours.
3. Once done, allow it to stay for 5 minute then pour this mixture into a casserole dish, lined with parchment paper.
4. Keep it in the refrigerator for 30 minutes to chill until it is firm.
5. Slice and serve.

### Nutrients

Calories: 65          Fats: 5g          Sodium: 21mg

Carbs: 2g          Proteins: 1g          Sugar: 8.2g

# Super Fudgy Slow Cooker Brownies

**Serves: 6**

**Prep Time: 5 mins**

A surprisingly healthy twist to a chocolate fudge would be the addition of bok choy to its basic ingredients.   That is right, the bok choy, a juicy green Asian vegetable is added to the fudge to make it more nourishing and delicious than ever.

## Ingredients

- 1 (5 count) package Jade Asian Greens Baby Shanghai Bok Choy
- 2 tablespoons water
- 1/2 teaspoon salt
- 1 cup almond flour
- 1/2 cup cocoa powder
- 1/2 cup sugar or granulated sweetener of choice
- 1 teaspoon baking powder
- 1/2 teaspoon espresso powder
- 2 large eggs
- 1/3 cup coconut oil, melted
- 1 teaspoon vanilla extract
- 1/3 cup chocolate chips (optional)

## Directions

1. Grease a 6 quart slow cooker with olive oil. Keep it aside.
2. Trim the stems of bok choy and boil it in saucepan with salted water for 5 minutes.
3. Once boiled transfer the bok choy to a blender and puree it well.
4. Mix espresso powder, cocoa powder, almond flour, sweetener and baking powder in a large bowl.

5. Add eggs, bok choy puree coconut oil and vanilla extract to the flour mixture and whisk well.

6. Fold in chocolate chips then pour this mixture into the slow cooker.

7. Cook for 3 to 4 hours on low setting.

8. Once done, allow it to cool and slice it into small squares.

9. Serve and enjoy.

## Nutrition

Calories: 187

Fats: 20.8g

Sodium: 5mg

Carbs: 10.33g

Proteins: 6.68g

Sugar: 11.3g

# Grain-Free Low-Carb Sugar-Free Granola

**Serves: 6**

**Prep Time: 10 mins**

You might have tried variety of granolas at home, but this grain free granola is a perfect alternative for a keto diet. It is made out of crunchy mix of all our favorite nuts including almonds, walnuts, hazelnuts and pecans. Mix it all up with pumpkin seeds, sunflower seeds and coconut shreds to add more comforting flavor.

## Ingredients
- 1/3 cup coconut oil
- 1 teaspoon vanilla extract
- 1 teaspoon vanilla stevia
- 1/2 cup raw almonds
- 1/2 cup walnuts
- 1/2 cup pecans
- 1/2 cup hazelnuts
- 2 cups raw sunflower seeds and pumpkin seeds 1 cup each
- 1 cup unsweetened shredded coconut
- 1/2 cup Swerve sweetener
- 1 teaspoon ground cinnamon
- 1 teaspoon salt
- 1 cup whipped cream

## Directions
1. Grease the base of the slow cooker with coconut oil.
2. Add stevia, vanilla extract, seeds, nuts and coconut to the cooker. Mix well.
3. Mix cinnamon with salt and swerve in a bowl and pour it over the nuts mixture.

4. Cover the lid and cook on low for 2 hours. Give occasional stirs after every 30 minutes.
5. Transfer the cooked granula over a baking sheet and spread it out to cool.
6. Serve with whipped cream on top or store in a sealed container for later use.

**Nutrients**

Calories: 337          Fats: 31.6g          Sodium: 3mg
Carbs: 8.7g          Proteins: 7.9g          Sugar: 18.9g

# Low-Sugar and Gluten-Free Slow Cooker Blueberry Crisp

**Serves: 4**

**Prep Time:   5mins**

Blueberry crispy is complete dessert which has the juicy mixture of fresh blueberries and the crunchy mixture of oats and walnuts. To experience a more flavorsome taste, serve this low carb crispy with cream or ice cream toppings.

## Ingredients

- 24 oz. frozen blueberries, about 5 cups
- 1 1/2 cups rolled oats, coarsely ground in food processor or bowl attachment of an immersion blender
- 1/4 cup melted butter
- 1/4 cup melted coconut oil
- 1 cup coarsely chopped pecans or walnuts
- 3/4 cup blanched almond flour
- 3/4 teaspoon salt
- 1/4 cup Stevia-in-the-Raw Granulated Sweetener or Monk Fruit Sweetener
- 2 tablespoons brown sugar

## Directions

1. Grease a slow cooker with a nonstick spray and add 5 cups of blueberries to it.
2. Mix nuts with ground oats, salt, stevia, almond flour, sugar, butter and sweetener in a bowl.
3. Spread this mixture over the layers of blueberries in the cooker.
4. Cover and cook on high for 3 to 4 hours.
5. Once done, bake the crispy in a preheated oven at 400 F.

6. Serve warm with ice cream or whipped cream on top.

## Nutrition

| | | |
|---|---|---|
| Calories: 202 | Fats: 12g | Sodium: 21mg |
| Carbs: 11.7g | Proteins: 0.8g | Sugar: 2.3g |

# Slow Cooker Low Carb Maple Custard

**Serves: 4**

**Prep Time: 10mins**

Prepare a maple and cinnamon custard using your slow cooker. It is completely gluten free and offers a low carb alternative for an ordinary custard. Cook the mixture of good cream and milk with the essence of cinnamon to add a strong taste.

## Ingredients

- 2 eggs
- 1 cup heavy cream horizon organic
- 1/2 cup whole milk horizon organic
- 1/4 cup Sukrin gold or another sugar-free brown sugar substitute
- 1 teaspoon maple extract
- 1/4 teaspoon salt
- 1/2 teaspoon cinnamon

## Directions

1. Mix all the ingredients together in a mixer and blend well on medium speed until combined.
2. Grease 4oz. ramekins and pour the batter into each upto ¾ full.
3. Place the ramekins in the slow cooker.
4. Cover the lid and cook for 2 hours on high.
5. Once done, remove the ramekins from the cooker and allow to cool for 1 hour.
6. Refrigerate for 2 hours then serve with whipped cream and cinnamon powder on top.

## Nutrition

Calories: 190

Fats: 10g

Sodium: 144mg

Carbs: 2g

Proteins: 4g

Sugar: 1g

# Sugar-Free Pumpkin Pie Bars

**Serves: 12**

**Prep Time: 5mins**

These pumpkin pie bars will make you popular among all but its balanced mixture of pumpkin puree, cream, pumpkin spice and cream. Together with eggs, the filling of the bars gives a mouthwatering flavor which is more enhanced by that crust of shredded coconut, cocoa powder and seeds.

## Ingredients

Crust:

- 3/4 cup unsweetened shredded coconut
- 1/4 cup unsweetened cocoa powder
- 1/2 cup raw unsalted sunflower seeds or sunflower seed flour
- 1/4 teaspoon salt
- 1/4 cup Swerve
- 4 tablespoons butter softened

Filling:

- 1 29 ounce can pumpkin puree
- 1 cup heavy cream
- 6 eggs
- 1/2 teaspoon salt
- 1 tablespoon vanilla extract
- 1 tablespoon pumpkin pie spice
- 1 teaspoon cinnamon liquid stevia
- 1 teaspoon pure stevia extract

## Directions

1. Add all the ingredients for the crust into a food processor and grind until fine crumbs.
2. Grease the base of a slow cooker and pour the grinded mixture into it.
3. Press the mixture firmly to form a uniform crust.
4. Add the ingredients for the filing to a mixer and blend well.
5. Fold in chocolate chips and pour this batter over the crust.
6. Cover the lid and cook for 3 hours on low.
7. Once done, allow it to cool for 30 minutes then refrigerator for 3 hours.
8. Slice and serve.

## Nutrients

| | | |
|---|---|---|
| Calories: 151 | Fats: 12.4g | Sodium: 155mg |
| Carbs: 6.2g | Proteins: 5.4g | Sugar: 1.8g |

# Slow Cooker Raspberry Cream Cheese Coffee Cake

**Serves: 12**

**Prep Time: 10 mins**

Who doesn't like a bite full of juicy raspberries and when they are incorporated into a nice coffee cheese cream cake, the temptation gets doubled. The cake is simple to cook when there is slow cooker available. Just whisk the basic ingredients together and top it with raspberries then bake slowly on low.

## Ingredients

Cake Batter:

- 1 1/4 almond flour
- 1/2 cup Swerve Sweetener
- 1/4 cup coconut flour
- 1/4 cup Organic Valley Vanilla Fuel Protein Powder
- 1 1/2 teaspoons baking powder
- 1/4 teaspoon salt
- 3 large eggs
- 6 tablespoons Organic Valley Pasture Butter melted
- 2/3 cup water
- 1/2 teaspoon vanilla extract

Filling:

- 8 ounces Organic Valley cream cheese
- 1/3 cup powdered Swerve Sweetener
- 1 large egg
- 2 tablespoons Organic Valley whipping cream
- 1 1/2 cup fresh raspberries

## Directions

1. Grease a 6 quart slow cooker and keep it aside.
2. Mix all the ingredients for the cake and keep them aside.
3. Beat the ingredients of the filling in a separate bowl and keep it aside.
4. First pour the two third of the cake batter into the slow cooker then top it with layer of cream cheese mixture.
5. Add raspberries over this layer then dot the remaining batter over the cream layer.
6. Cover the lid and on low for 3 to 4 hours.
7. Once done, remove the cake from the cooker and refrigerate well before serving.
8. Slice, serve and enjoy.

## Nutrition

Calories: 239

Fats: 19.18g

Sodium: 16mg

Carbs: 6.95g

Proteins: 7.54g

Sugar: 10.1g

# Low Carb Blueberry Lemon Custard Cake

**Serves: 12**

**Prep Time: 5mins**

Blueberry with lemon, here is combination which your taste buds will remember for quite some time. The custard cake has mild sour and an earthly sweet taste which is aided by the lemon zest and cream. Blueberries are sprinkled over the batter to keep them fresh from the first bite Uptil the last one.

## Ingredients

- 6 eggs separated
- 1/2 cup Bob's Red Mill Coconut Flour
- 2 teaspoons lemon zest
- 1/3 cup lemon juice
- 1 teaspoon lemon liquid stevia
- 1/2 cup Swerve sweetener
- 1/2 teaspoon salt
- 2 cups light cream
- 1/2 cup fresh blueberries

## Direction

1. Add egg whites to a mixer and beat well until foamy. Keep them aside.
2. Beat yolks with all the other ingredients except blueberries.
3. Gradually stir in the foamy egg white mixture. Mix well.
4. Grease a slow cooker and pour this batter into it.
5. Top the batter with blueberries.
6. Cover the lid and cook for 3 hours on low setting.
7. Once done, allow the cake to cool then refrigerate for 2 hours or more.

8. Top with whipped cream and serve.

**Nutrition**

Calories: 140

Fats: 9.2g

Sodium: 167mg

Carbs: 7.3g

Proteins: 3.9g

Sugar: 3.5g

# Slow Cooker Chocolate Cake

**Serves: 10**

**Prep Time: 10mins**

A low carb chocolate cake does exist in the real word. But to make this happen, you need following basic ingredients which are readily available in the market. Just use simple mixing techniques and cook it well in your slow cooker with complete ease and confidence.

## Ingredients

- 1 cup plus 2 tablespoons almond flour
- 1/2 cup Swerve, Granular
- 1/2 cup cocoa powder
- 3 tablespoons unflavored whey protein powder
- 1 1/2 teaspoons baking powder
- 1/4 teaspoon salt
- 3 large eggs
- 6 tablespoons butter, melted
- 2/3 cup unsweetened almond milk
- 3/4 teaspoon vanilla extract
- 1/3 cup sugar-free chocolate chips

## Directions

1. Grease a 6 quart slow cooker and keep it aside.
2. Mix all the dry ingredients together in a bowl.
3. Whisk eggs with butter, vanilla and almond milk in a bowl and stir in the dry mixture.
4. Mix well then fold in the chocolate chips.
5. Pour this batter into the cooker and cover the lid to cook on low for 2 to 2.5 hours.

6. Once done, allow the cake to cook for 30 minutes then slice it into pieces.
7. Serve warm and enjoy.
8. Grease the insert of a 6 quart slow cooker well.

**Nutrition**

Calories: 144

Fats: 16.97g

Sodium: 29mg

Carbs: 8.4g

Proteins: 7.37g

Sugar: 11.4g

# Slow Cooker Lemon Custard

**Serves: 4**

**Prep Time: 10mins**

A slow cooker lemon custard is a nice creamy and milky extract of lemon zest and lemon juice which cooked together with egg yolks, vanilla extracts and whipped cream. For best flavor refrigerate well and chill before serving then enjoy as after dinner, weekend night special dessert.

## Ingredients

- 5 large egg yolks
- 1/4 cup freshly squeezed lemon juice
- 1 tablespoon lemon zest
- 1 teaspoon vanilla extract
- 1/2 teaspoon liquid stevia
- 2 cups whipping cream or coconut cream
- Lightly sweetened whipped cream or whipped coconut cream

## Directions

1. Whisk egg yolks with lemon zest, vanilla, stevia and lemon juice in a bowl.
2. Add heavy cream and whisk again well. Divide the mixture into 4 ramekins.
3. Place the ramekins in the slow cooker and cover the lid to cooker for 3 hours on Low.
4. Once done, remove the ramekins from the cooker and allow them to cool.
5. Refrigerate for about 3 hours then serve with whipped cream on top.

## Nutrition

Calories: 319        Fats: 30g        Sodium: 11mg

Carbs: 3g        Proteins: 7g        Sugar: 1.2g

# Conclusion

The easiest way to a healthy life style is following the ketogenic diet. Burning fats instead of carbohydrates certainly helps in a lot is weight loss and maintaining your physical health. A slow cooker is the best method to cook you ketogenic food and conveniently achieve a healthy lifestyle.

And on top of it, one of our biggest challenges in eating well is — time- it is so easy to fast food and go after a long day, but the slow cooker is our friend. All you have to do is pop your ingredients into the slow cooker at night and wake up to a beautiful breakfast or lunch. In the same vein, you pop your ingredients for dinner in the morning and in the eve is waiting for you delicious magical stuff.

When you fuel your body with the best foods, you are taking yourself to a whole new level of cognition, wellness and a body that just won't quit. Welcome to your amazing new life of eating well and loving it too.

Made in the USA
Lexington, KY
17 September 2018